Winning Over
Diabetes

Prevention through
Understanding

Dr Rita Malik & Dr T.K. Malik

ISBN: 1494875926
ISBN-13: 9781494875923

40,46,77,121.
TXu 1-895-537 effective date of registrations:
December 13, 2013

This book is dedicated to our grandchildren:
Gautam Malik, Riya Malik, and Anya Malik.

ACKNOWLEDGMENTS

We thank our sons, Niten Malik and Chetan Malik. Niten inspired us to write this book and helped us all the way. Chetan helped in getting all relevant books and literature from the library and made it available to us.
We thank the team at CreateSpace for their efforts to make this book a success story.

CONTENTS

explains insulin's mode of action, maintenance of blood glucose levels, and regulation of insulin secretion.

PART 2

Awareness of diabetes is exceedingly low; most people are not familiar with the presenting features. This chapter describes the modes of presentation.

What is diabetes mellitus, and what are its variants? What is the role of heredity in types of diabetes? What is insulin resistance? What does it imply? And is there anything we can do about it?

How can you know you have diabetes and be sure it is not something else? This chapter provides the diagnostic criteria of the World Health Organization and discusses how to monitor blood sugar levels.

This chapter describes the precautions to take and rules to follow when diabetes is associated with pregnancy. The perverse fascination with alcoholic drinks and relentless decline in simple living has driven people away from nature and made them prey to ailments, even more so the diabetic.

This chapter describes the role of the cardiovascular system in preserving the internal environment of the body (the fluid that surrounds and bathes the individual cells). It elaborates on the changes that take place in the body when a person develops diabetes, the consequences, and the development of complications.

The morbidity and mortality of the complications from diabetes are profound.

PART 3

The secret to health is preventing disease; this chapter discusses the necessary measures.

This chapter discusses type 1 and type 2 diabetes in children, obesity (a prime cause of disease), and the responsibilities of parents.

A scientist announced that the "gene proposes and environment disposes": the environment exposes what we have inherited. Our health depends to a great extent on our activities.

Tackling obesity is a million-dollar question. This chapter discusses the causes and management of obesity.

At times circumstances are such that stress is inevitable. This chapter discusses the generation of stress and how to negate it.

INTRODUCTION

For time immemorial infectious diseases such as malaria, tuberculosis, and smallpox have posed challenges to the human population. They continue to do so in third world countries. However, diabetes, cancer, and heart disease have assumed positions of deep concern for the human race.

Obesity is associated with diabetes. The cost of diabetic health care runs into millions of dollars. The burden of being overweight is indeed heavy.

Some sects of society, such as common laborers, hermits, nuns, and monks, follow simple living. The saints and hermits of ancient India had simple and unique lifestyles. They lived in mountains; had their dwellings near streams, rivers, and springs; derived their food from nature; and spent most of their time meditating. Yoga was an essential part of their lifestyle, and they lived long, healthy lives.

Such a lifestyle may not be possible in today's world. The increased consumption of fast food and processed food and the relative lack of exercise are the root causes of many human ailments. One such ailment is diabetes (the "sugar problem," in layman's language).

I have many friends and relatives who suffer from diabetes, yet surprisingly only a few of them take their disease seriously. Most of them are casual or even reckless about their predicaments and become serious about their disease only when serious complications hit them. A friend of mine continued to abuse alcohol and indulge in gourmet meals in spite of repeated warnings. He ultimately died of kidney failure at the age of forty.

Another, a lady of forty, is a close relative of ours. She is not bothered by her high fasting blood sugar level of 291 mg/dl, but she is worried about her eighty-two-year-old mother, who has vertigo. Normal fasting glucose level is at or below 100 mg percent.

The purpose of this book is to make diabetic patients aware of the debilitating complications that may afflict them and how to avoid such conditions.

The book provides an easy-to-understand yet comprehensive overview of what happens to a person suffering from diabetes. It explains the attitudes that precipitate diabetes in certain ethnic and genetic settings. It helps the reader to better understand this complex disease and how it affects every organ, and it empowers diabetics to understand the changes they must make in their day-to-day lives.

We all have philosophies by which we conduct our lives. They determine our lines of thinking and help us decide what is right or wrong. This book details a philosophy that helps regulate the lifestyle of a person suffering from diabetes. It does not outline a treatment, which should always be determined by your treating doctor. It is merely a theme that will help you help yourself.

The first part of the book introduces the disease and details its historical aspects. It describes the prevalence of the disease and how the body functions normally.

The second part details the common modes of presentation and the types, causes, and complications of diabetes.

The third part describes how a predisposed individual might avoid the disease and discusses how to manage the disease once it becomes manifest. With this condition all the organs of the body are affected, so readers should know how best to prevent serious complications. A portion is devoted to obesity and innovations in the field of diabetes.

The book also gives descriptions of home remedies and herbs and explains the health benefits of natural foods. The last section describes tasteful Indian recipes that are good for diabetics.

PART 1

CHAPTER 1

Diabetes Is No Disaster

I know nothing except the fact of my ignorance.
—Socrates

The early phase of diabetes is impaired glucose tolerance, when blood glucose levels are between normal and diabetic levels. This is the stage when efforts can be made to prevent or delay diabetes. It is silent at that stage; later it becomes manifest and then eats away the body like rust. It depletes the body and devastates every vital organ, becoming a bitter life partner. However, you can turn back the clock and start on the path of a healthy, long life. The secret is to make sensible, workable changes in your lifestyle.

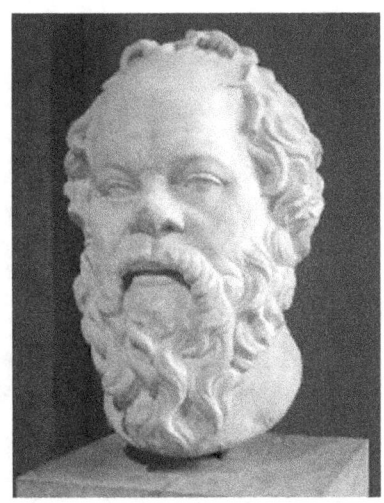

Socrates[1]

Individual Reaction to Diabetes

When a person is first diagnosed as diabetic, the initial feeling is alarm, shock, or depression. The sinking feeling gives way to reconciliation and acceptance. While some patients gear up to face the challenge, others fail to perceive the gravity of the situation and remain indifferent and careless; perhaps they do not know about the consequences of the disorder. Some are under the misconception that their disease is mild, and they take liberties. Diabetes is no disaster, but it should be treated seriously.

There Is No Need for Denial or Despair

What matters most at this stage is the person's attitude, determination, and motivation to face the disease and make the necessary lifestyle changes.

Some famous people who had diabetes are Ernest Hemingway, H. G. Wells, Elizabeth Taylor, and Elvis Presley.[3]

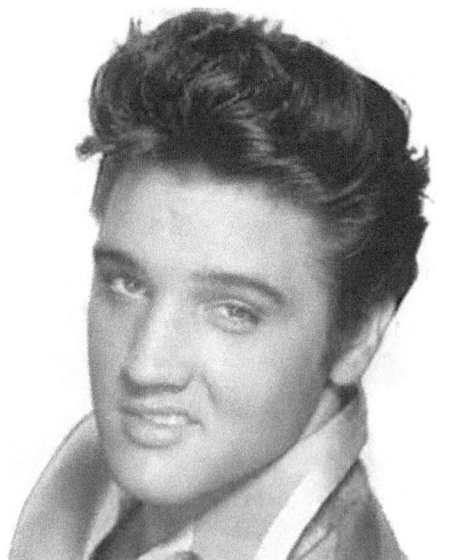

Elvis Presley[2]

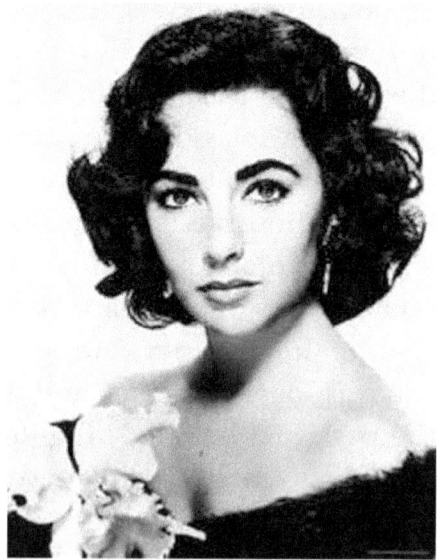

Elizabeth Taylor[4]

These luminaries did wonders in their lifetime, so why can't you and I?

The discovery of diabetes should make patients lead more disciplined lives, leading to better quality of life. They must realign their lifestyles and activities. By doing so they might delay the process of aging and the onset of complications.

They need the support of family and friends because diabetes is a lifelong disorder with many complications. The patients must understand all facets of the disease and take the necessary measures to lead healthy lives.[6]

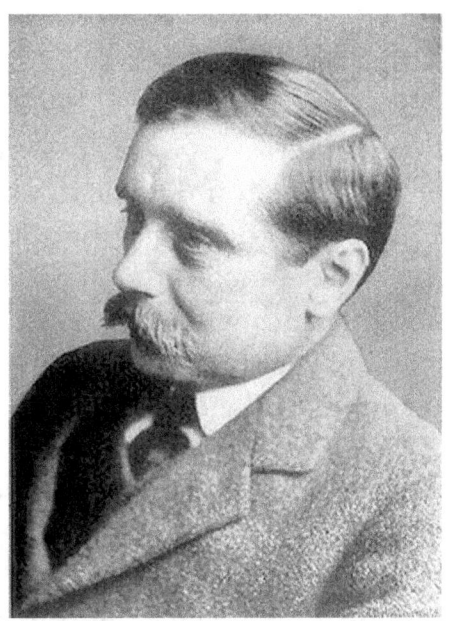

H. G. Wells[5]

The human mind is a marvelous thing. It can achieve any objective it sets its mind to. The mind can look after the body, but to do so it needs to be enlightened with knowledge. The functions of the body are intricately designed, delicately interwoven, and finely tuned. A small defect can put the entire machinery in chaos.

This is true of diabetes more than any other disorder. The discipline of medicine is a steadily growing knowledge base that guides scientists to make concrete improvements in the management, survival, and the quality of life of diabetics. In this age of science, explorative insights and research initiatives have brought an era of hope. Knowledge is imperative for managing this ailment under the guidance of a medical professional.

Managing Diabetes

Diabetes is a lifelong disorder that is markedly affected by variations in diet, exercise, infection, and stress.[7,8] These factors must be addressed on daily basis, and the patient is the person best equipped to deal with the situation. A thorough knowledge of the disease, including how it alters normal body functions and what its acute and chronic complications are, enables patients to take better care of it. Awareness and better health care improve the long-term outlook of patients with this disease.

Because managing diabetes is so intimately linked to food, information about food, nutrition, the scientific base of biochemistry, physiology,[9] and pathogenesis helps patients understand this disorder. (*Pathos* refers to an abnormal state, and *genesis* signifies generation; hence *pathogenesis* means "the development of an abnormal state.")

The following chapters explore all aspects of the disease and its management. Each chapter deals with one aspect of the condition. All the chapters combined weave into a comprehensive text, and a complete picture of the diabetic state and its management emerges.

CHAPTER 2

Diabetes through the Ages

Those who fail to read history are destined to suffer from repetition of mistakes.
- George Santayana

This chapter pays homage to the great scientists who made remarkable discoveries and revealed the evolution of the disease from diagnosis to management.

In Ayurvedic (ancient Indian) medicine, diabetes is mentioned. The oldest known Ayurvedic texts are the *Sushruta Sa hit* and the *Charaka Sa hit*. These classical Sanskrit texts are among the foundational and formally compiled works of Ayurveda, the science of traditional ancient Indian medicine; the drugs are derived from plants.

As far back as 1000 BC, Sushruta, an Indian surgeon, was the first to identify diabetes and link it to something being wrong in the blood. In the late nineteenth century, two German scientists, Joseph von Mering and Oskar Minkowski, made landmark discoveries, and later Frederick Banting and Charles Best discovered insulin.

Continuing research has led to the formation of synthetic human insulin. Today gene mapping, genetic engineering, and pancreatic transplantation are at the frontier of research.

The Ancient History of Diabetes

Diabetes has a worldwide distribution and is prevalent in both developing and developed countries. It has afflicted many over the ages, cutting across geographic and racial barriers. It was recognized more than two thousand years ago; the ancient Indians, Chinese, Romans, and Greeks knew it. The Romans found that patients who suffered from this condition passed urine having a sweet taste (the Latin word for *sweet* is *mellitus*). The Greeks found that such patients passed urine as rapidly as they drank water, as if it was being siphoned out (the Greek word for *siphon* is *diabetes*). Hence the disease assumed a unique nomenclature straddling two civilizations: it was called diabetes mellitus.

Ayurvedic literature referenced a disease resembling diabetes as far back as 1000 BC. *Prameha* is a condition where urine is passed excessively. In Sanskrit the prefix *pra* means "excessive in frequency and quantity," and *meha* means "watering." In Sanskrit texts prameha is further classified, and one type is referred to as *madhumeha*. The prefix *madhu* means sweet, and so the word *madhumeha* refers to a disease more closely resembling diabetes mellitus.

Some important earlier discoveries include the following:
- In 1500 BC Papyrus Ebrs, an Egyptian, used remedies for patients who were passing too much urine.
- Arabian writers translated information about diabetes from ancient Indian texts.

- Greek physicians in 275–230 BC diagnosed diabetes and associated it with weakness of the kidneys, loss of water, and dehydration. They used rockfish, the juice of knotgrass, and potherbs such as lettuce as remedies.
- Sushrata's works (1622–1675) describe diabetes as a disease of the blood due to hormonal changes.
- In 1798 John Rolls showed that diabetics have excess sugar in the blood.
- L. Trube (1816–1876) showed a link between carbohydrate intake and the presence of sugar in urine.

In the late nineteenth century, as Western science made giant leaps in research and exploration, vital breakthroughs were achieved.

Diabetes in Ayurveda

Ayurveda is the science of ancient Indian medicine. The cause, pathogenesis, and treatments of diabetes mellitus mentioned in Ayurvedic texts are astonishingly similar to the modern concepts of diabetes. The two types of madhumeha (lean diabetic and the obese diabetic, in Vedic classification) are strikingly similar to modern type 1 and type 2 diabetes. Similarly there are references to congenital variants: *sahaja prameha* (due to a defective seed [gene]) and *apathyanimitthaja prameha* (due to overeating and wrong eating habits).

Two stalwarts of ancient Indian medicine, Charaka and Sushrata, wrote extensively on madhumeha. Charaka was an able and renowned physician; Sushrata was an equally competent surgeon and was the first to diagnose diabetes. Both have many treaties to their credit, which were called *samhitas.*

Their texts refer to diabetes as *madhumeha,* and it is an appropriate term. Sushruta devoted a complete chapter to the treatment of madhumeha in his book *Samhitas.* He considered it a more complicated form of prameha. At that time, when modern investigations were not known, diabetes insipidus, an endocrinal disorder in which excessive urine is passed, was considered a distinct type of prameha.

The Discovery of Insulin

In 1889 two German scientists discovered that a dog whose pancreas had been removed passed sugar in its urine. Joseph von Mering and Oskar Minkowski proved that pancreatic secretion controlled the body's use of sugar. The hormone secreted by the pancreas is called insulin. Dr. Frederick Banting and Dr. Charles Best discovered insulin in 1921, and in 1923 John J. R. Macleod and Frederick Banting won the Nobel Prize in medicine for their work. Thirty years later Frederick Sanger defined the amino acid sequence of bovine insulin and received the Nobel Prize in chemistry. This pioneering research led to the formation of synthetic human insulin.

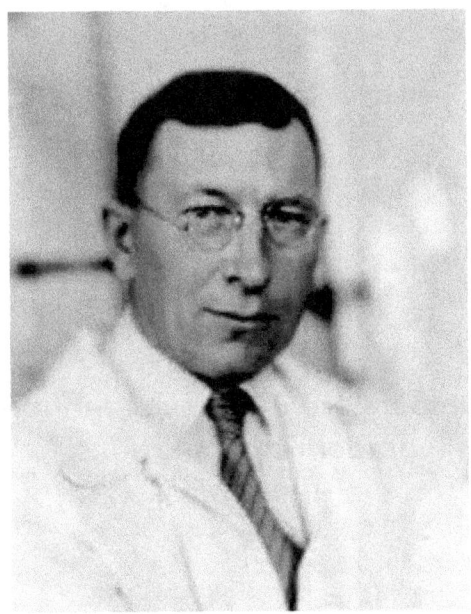

Frederick Banting[10]

CHAPTER 3

Stark Statistics

*The numbers are increasing and touching
epidemic proportions.*
—Rita Malik

Statistics of disease help elucidate causative factors. By virtue of statistics, it has been ascertained that cigarette smoking is linked to lung cancer.

Statistics are not just numbers.[11] They are powerful tools that reveal the history of a disease, give insight into its evolution, and predict the future. This chapter describes the prevalence of diabetes based on geographic variance and ethnic, racial, and socioeconomic status. The data obtained throws light on the etiology and evolution of the disease. It also gives the prevalence rate of complications. The effects of rich, fatty foods and a sedentary lifestyle are also discussed.

Worldwide Incidence of Diabetes
It is estimated that about 250 million persons around the world have diabetes. Per projected estimates the global prevalence is likely to touch the 360 million mark by the year 2030. In America there are about twenty-six million people with diabetes, and the

number is rapidly increasing. Of these, 1.4 million have type 1 diabetes, and the remaining mostly have type 2. For all ages 90 percent of people with diabetes have type 2, but for those older than forty-five, virtually all people with diabetes have type 2. Type 1 is one of the most common chronic diseases in children in the United States, and its incidence is increasing around the world. For all ages the incidence of diagnosed diabetes is equal to or slightly higher in women.

Between 1990 and 2001, US government surveys showed diabetes cases almost doubling among people between the ages of thirty and fifty, and the number increased by half in those between the ages of eighteen and twenty-nine.

Geographic Incidence

There is remarkable variation in the geographic incidence of diabetes. The incidence of type 1 is 0.7 per 100,000 in Shanghai, China, while it is twenty-six times greater in whites in Allegheny County, Pennsylvania (18.2 per 100,000) and is more than fifty times greater in Finland (35.3 per 100,000).

India may be the diabetes capital of world. The World Health Organization (WHO) projects India to have the fastest growing number of diabetics. In the year 2000, a survey carried out by the Indian Council of Medical Research (ICMR) showed that India is home to approximately thirty-two million diabetic patients in a population of more than one billion. Worse still it is estimated this figure will grow to fifty-seven million by 2025.

Research conducted in Madras on twenty-six thousand people who were older than twenty showed that at least 12 percent of them had diabetes. About half of the affected people suffered from hypertension but did not know they had the disease. The research director said, "Awareness levels are appallingly low."

Worldwide Prevalence of Diabetes, 2000–2030

Diabetes is a global problem with devastating social and economic impacts. It is expected that the number will increase to more than 380 million by 2025.

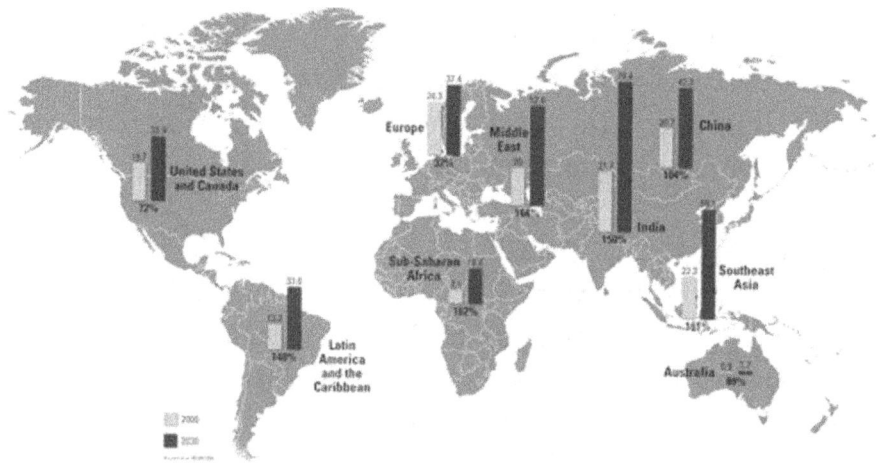

Global Diabetes Statistics[12]

The Global Burden[13]

- The number of people with type 2 diabetes is increasing in every country.
- Eighty percent of people with diabetes live in low- and middle-income countries.
- Most people with diabetes are between forty and fifty-nine years old.
- Roughly 183 million people (50 percent) with diabetes are undiagnosed.
- Diabetes caused 4.6 million deaths in 2011.

- Diabetes caused at least $465 billion in health-care expenditures in 2011 (11 percent of total health-care expenditures in adults twenty to seventy-nine years old).
- Roughly 78,000 children develop type 1 diabetes every year.

Total prevalence of diabetes[14,15]
- Approximately 25.8 million children and adults in the United States—8.3 percent of the population—have diagnosed diabetes.
- Undiagnosed: 7 million people
- Prediabetes*: 79 million people
- New cases: 1.9 million diagnosed in people age twenty and older in 2010.

  *Prediabetes is the phase where blood sugar levels are higher than normal but below those in diabetics.

In contrast to the 2007 National Diabetes Fact Sheet, which used fasting glucose data to estimate undiagnosed diabetes and prediabetes, the 2011 National Diabetes Fact Sheet used both fasting glucose and HbA1c levels to derive estimates for undiagnosed diabetes and prediabetes. These tests were chosen because they are most frequently used in clinical practice. Prediabetes is a phase of impaired glucose tolerance. HbA1c is the test that gives the average glucose level in the previous three months. HbA1c is complex, formed by a combination of hemoglobin and blood glucose.

Number of people younger than twenty years who have diabetes:
- 215,000, or 0.26 percent of all people in this age group.
- About one in every four hundred children and adolescents.

Number of people age twenty or older:
- 25.6 million, or 11.3 percent of all people in this age group.

Number of people age sixty-five or older:
- 10.9 million, or 26.9 percent of all people in this age group.

Men:
- 13.0 million, or 11.8 percent of men age twenty or older.

Women:
- 12.6 million, or 10.8 percent of women age twenty or older.

Race and Ethnic Differences in Prevalence of Diagnosed Diabetes

After adjusting for population age differences, 2007–2009 national survey data for people diagnosed with diabetes age twenty or older include the following prevalence by race/ethnicity:
- 7.1 percent of non-Hispanic whites.
- 8.4 percent of Asian Americans.
- 12.6 percent of non-Hispanic blacks.
- 11.8 percent of Hispanics.

Hispanics' rates were as follows:
- 7.6 percent of Cubans.
- 13.3 percent of Mexican Americans.
- 13.8 percent of Puerto Ricans.

Morbidity and Mortality

In 2007 diabetes was listed as the underlying cause on 71,382 death certificates and listed as a contributing factor on an additional 160,022 death certificates. This means diabetes contributed to a total of 231,404 deaths.

Complications

Heart Disease and Stroke

The blood vessels of the heart and brain get occluded, resulting in heart disease and stroke.[16]

- In 2004 heart disease was noted on 68 percent of diabetes-related death certificates among people age sixty-five or older.
- In 2004 stroke was noted on 16 percent of diabetes-related death certificates among people age sixty-five or older.
- Adults with diabetes have heart-disease death rates two to four times higher than adults without diabetes.
- The risk of stroke is two to four times higher among people with diabetes.

High Blood Pressure

- From 2005 to 2008, of adults age twenty or older with self-reported diabetes, 67 percent had blood pressure greater than or equal to 130/90 mmHg (systolic/diastolic) or used prescription medications for hypertension.[17] Normal systolic blood pressure ranges between 90 and 130 mmHg and diastolic between 60 and 90mmHg.

Blindness

- Diabetes is the leading cause of new cases of blindness among adults age twenty to seventy-four.

- From 2005 to 2008, 4.2 million people (28.5 percent) with diabetes age forty or older had diabetic retinopathy, and of these almost 0.7 million (4.4 percent of those with diabetes) had advanced diabetic retinopathy that could lead to severe vision loss.[18]

Kidney Disease
- Diabetes is the leading cause of kidney failure, accounting for 44 percent of new cases in 2008.[19]
- In 2008 in the United States, 48,374 people with diabetes began treatment for end-stage kidney disease.
- In 2008 a total of 202,290 people in the United States with end-stage kidney disease due to diabetes were living on chronic dialysis or with transplanted kidneys.

Nervous System Disease (Neuropathy)
- 60 to 70 percent of people with diabetes have mild to severe forms of nervous system damage.[20]

Amputation
- More than 60 percent of nontraumatic lower-limb amputations occur in people with diabetes.
- In 2006 about 65,700 nontraumatic lower-limb amputations were performed on people with diabetes.

The Cost of Diabetes
- $174 billion: total cost of diagnosed diabetes in the United States in 2007.
- $116 billion went to direct medical costs.
- $58 billion went to indirect costs (disability, work loss, premature mortality).

After adjusting for population age and sex differences, the average medical expenditures among people with diagnosed diabetes were 2.3 times higher than what expenditures would be in the absence of diabetes.

The American Diabetes Association (ADA) has created a diabetes cost calculator that takes national data on the cost of diabetes and provides estimates at the state and congressional district levels. Factoring in the additional costs of undiagnosed diabetes, prediabetes, and gestational diabetes brings the total cost of diabetes in the United States in 2007 to $218 billion,[21] including
- $18 billion for people with undiagnosed diabetes;
- $25 billion for people with prediabetes; and
- $623 million for people with gestational diabetes.

Diabetes and Impaired Glucose Tolerance (IGT)

Diabetes mellitus is one of the most common non-communicable diseases (NCDs) globally. It is the fourth or fifth leading cause of death in most high-income countries, and there is substantial evidence that it is epidemic in many economically developing and newly industrialized countries. It is undoubtedly one of the most challenging health problems in the twenty-first century.

The number of studies describing the possible causes and distribution of diabetes over the last twenty years has been extraordinary. These studies continue to confirm that low- and middle-income countries face the greatest burdens of diabetes. However, many governments and public-health planners remain largely unaware of the current magnitude or, more important, the potential for increases in diabetes and its serious complications in their countries.

Population-based diabetes studies consistently show that a substantial proportion of those found to have diabetes had not been previously diagnosed. Many people remain undiagnosed largely because there are few symptoms during the early years of type 2 diabetes, or they may not recognize symptoms as being related to diabetes.

In addition to diabetes, impaired glucose tolerance (IGT), in which the blood glucose level is higher than normal but not as high as in diabetes, is a major public-health problem. People with IGT have a higher risk of developing diabetes as well as an increased risk of cardiovascular disease.

Prevalence and Projections

The International Diabetic Federation's (IDF's) *Diabetes Atlas* estimates the prevalence of diabetes mellitus and IGT for the years 2011 and 2030. Data are provided for 216 countries and territories grouped into the seven IDF regions: Africa, Europe, Middle East and North Africa, North America and the Caribbean, South and Central America, Southeast Asia, and the Western Pacific.

Full details of the methods used to generate the prevalence estimates for diabetes in adults and the proportion undiagnosed, including how the data sources were evaluated and processed, can be found in the methods paper published in the journal *Diabetes Research and Clinical Practice* and in the IDF's *Diabetes Atlas*.

Consider these sobering statistics from the US Department of Health and Human Services, Indian Health Service:

- 2.2 times higher: the likelihood of American Indians and Alaska Natives to have diabetes compared to non-Hispanic whites.
- 68 percent: the percent increase in diabetes from 1994 to 2004 in American Indian and Alaska Native youth age fifteen to nineteen.
- 95 percent: the percent of American Indians and Alaska Natives with diabetes who have type 2 diabetes (as opposed to type 1 diabetes).
- 30 percent: the estimated percent of American Indians and Alaska Natives who have prediabetes

American Indians and Alaska Natives are clearly at greater risk. Educate yourself on how to prevent type 2 diabetes if you don't have it now or how to treat it effectively if you've been diagnosed.

Racial Incidence

There are also racial and ethnic variations. It is possible that ethnic and familial clustering is a result of shared genes, shared behavior, and environmental risk factors. Type 1 is more common in whites and Hispanics as compared to African Americans and Mexican Americans. However, type 2 has a higher prevalence in African Americans, Mexican Americans, and Native Americans compared to non-Hispanic whites. Among the different people, the incidence is higher in African Americans, Hispanics, Asians, and Native Americans. It is estimated that about 25 percent of cases of diabetes occur in minorities in the United States.

Diabetes and Obesity

As affluence is increasing in poor countries like India and China, so is the incidence of diabetes. Diabetes is linked to obesity, which can be linked to a sedentary lifestyle and fast food, which is the fallout of growing affluence. As wealth flows into a family, the food becomes rich and fatty, and sedentary habits creep in, so individuals become obese and tend to get diabetes.[22]

Grim or smiling, obese Sumo wrestlers are part of good television and even trigger packed houses. The grim reality is that more than 40 percent of these Japanese wrestlers are diabetics, although the incidence of diabetes is low in Japan (approximately 3 percent). Japanese people who have migrated to the United States and adopted American eating habits have also increased their rates of incidence.

The Necessity of Timely Diagnosis

It is estimated that the number of undiagnosed cases of diabetes equals the diagnosed cases. The number of cases of people with IGT is even more than the undiagnosed cases of diabetes. The prevalence of people with IGT follows similar trends as those of people with non-insulin-dependent diabetes mellitus (NIDDM), and similar variations exist in racial and ethnic groups. In people age twenty to forty-four, the prevalence ranges from 5.5 percent in non-Hispanic whites to 10.8 percent in African Americans.

It is believed that about eight hundred thousand new cases of diabetes are diagnosed every year in America, and fifty-four thousand people die from diabetes-related causes. Many are diagnosed at the development of a complication, such as blindness.

Diabetes is a major risk factor for heart disease, stroke, and amputation. It shortens the life-span on average up to fifteen years and is the sixth leading cause of death. The risk of heart disease is two to four times more common in patients with diabetes, as is the risk of stroke. It is the leading cause of blindness and accounts for 40 percent of end-stage renal disease.

David Loshak, in his review in the *American Journal of Preventive Medicine,* indicated that nearly three-quarters of adult diabetics in the United States have hypertension, regardless of age, sex, and ethnic origin.[23] Patients can benefit from efforts to prevent and control it. Some estimates predict diabetes will affect 8.9 percent of the US population by the year 2025.

CHAPTER 4

Biochemistry

It is good to know about elements, for it is elementary in the understanding of anything worth its salt.
—Rita Malik

Physics and chemistry form the backbone of modern technology and have enabled man to land on the moon. A little knowledge of biochemistry (chemistry as it pertains to human biology or chemical reactions occurring in living cells) goes a long way in understanding the complexities of diabetes.

We eat, drink, sleep, and work and consider these matters of fact, but we are not aware of how the millions of cells that constitute our bodies work. In this chapter we learn how individual cells function so we can live. The foods we eat—namely fats, proteins, and carbohydrates—are complex compounds. In this chapter the structure of simple molecules is explained in a manner that leads to the understanding of complex molecules as well as lipoproteins (complexes of fats and proteins) that play significant roles in the geneses of many diseases.

The human body is composed of millions of microscopic units called cells. These cells derive their energy from a type of sugar called glucose. We know how kids get a boost of energy when they eat chocolate. Similarly the cells in the body get energy by using sugar. The process of using glucose is called metabolism, and diabetes affects metabolism.

Cells are made of elements found in nature. Two or more elements combine to form substances called compounds. These compounds are classified into two broad categories: inorganic and organic. The inorganic compounds include different types of salts such as sodium chloride (common salt) and sodium hydroxide, an alkali. Organic compounds are made of two common elements: carbon and hydrogen. Nutrients such as proteins, fats, and carbohydrates are examples of organic compounds.

The Composition of Cells

Water, a molecule made of hydrogen and oxygen, is an integral constituent of every cell of the body. It is also the basic constituent of blood and other fluids. It constitutes about 70 percent of the total body mass. Calcium and phosphates, along with other inorganic elements, form an integral part of the cells of the bones and teeth. Human blood, like the organs in the body, is made of cells. Among them are red blood cells, which help carry oxygen from the lungs to all parts of the body. Iron, another element, is a major inorganic component of the hemoglobin present in red blood cells. Copper, zinc, selenium, molybdenum, and other elements are important and found in varying quantities throughout the body. Some form integral constituents of the tissues, and some act as catalysts for many metabolic reactions. Read the label of a multivitamin bottle, and you will see some of these inorganic compounds and elements.

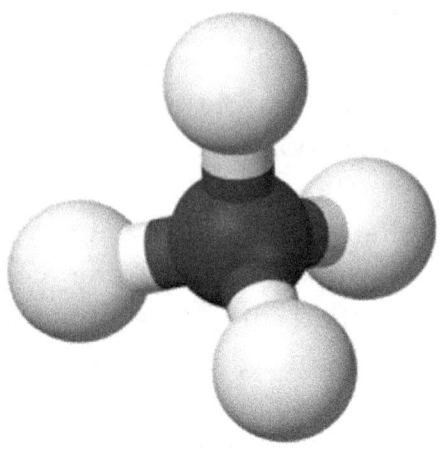

Methane and its derivatives[24]

This is a ball-and-stick model of the methane molecule, CH_4. Methane is part of a homologous series known as the alkanes, which contain single bonds only.

In organic chemistry, a hydrocarbon is an organic compound consisting entirely of hydrogen and carbon.

Proteins, fats, and carbohydrates are the three major organic compounds that constitute the human body. To understand the compounds that constitute any food we eat and play significant roles in our lives, let us learn the basic makeup of hydrocarbons. Organic compounds are derivatives of hydrocarbons,[25] which are compounds made of hydrogen and carbon. These elements are made of small particles called atoms. Each atom has its own combining capacity called its valence. Hydrogen has a single valence whereas carbon has four. Another way to describe this is that carbon has four hooks or hands and hydrogen has one. Carbon can hold four hydrogen atoms by virtue of its four hooks. One carbon atom combines with four hydrogen atoms to form a stable compound. The carbon atoms can also link with one another. They may link to one another to form simple and/or complex straight-chain compounds or join one another to form cyclic chains or ring-shaped molecules.

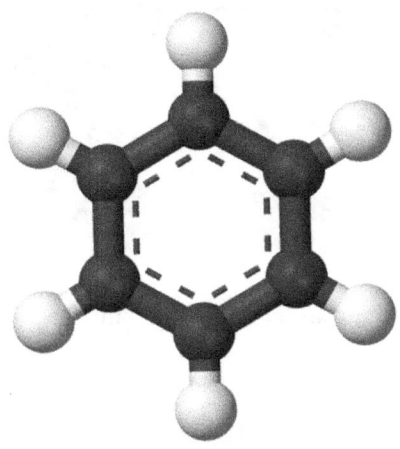

Benzene, a ring-shaped molecule[26]

A carbon having four valences can combine with four hydrogen atoms because each hydrogen atom has one valence to form straight-chain compounds (e.g., CH_4-methane and C_2H_6-ethane). These carbon atoms can combine with one another to form long straight-chain compounds (e.g., C-C-C-C). This four-chain carbon compound can combine with ten hydrogen atoms to form a stable molecule by saturating its remaining ten valences. The carbon atoms can also combine with one another to form cyclic compounds instead of straight-chain compounds, such as benzene.

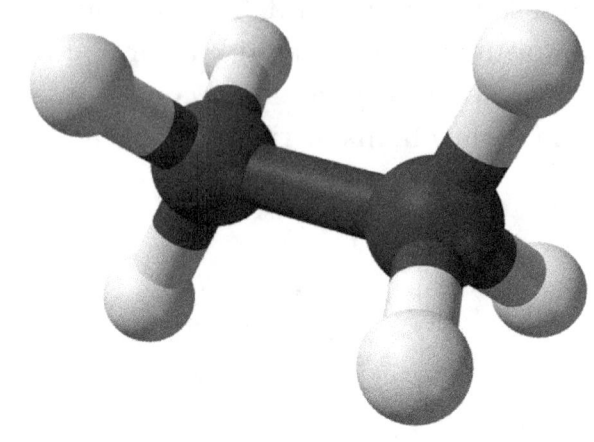

Ethane and its derivatives[27]

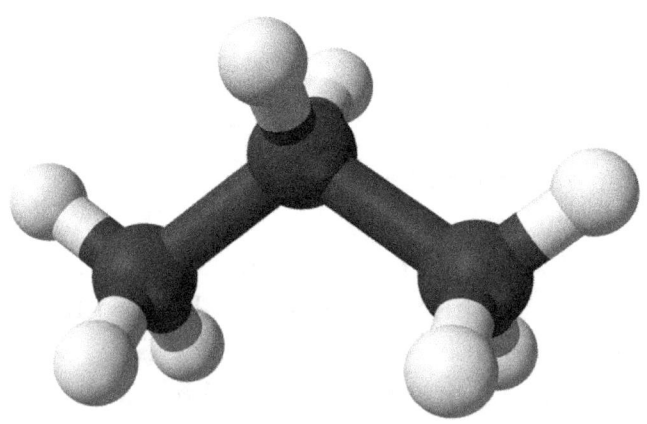

Propane and its derivatives[28]

If one atom of hydrogen in a hydrocarbon is replaced by an OH radical, called a hydroxyl group, which is also monovalent, an alcohol is formed (e.g., CH_3OH-methyl alcohol, a compound that is alkaline in nature). Methyl alcohol is an over-the-counter spirit found in pharmacies and used to clean wounds. When a hydrocarbon has multiple hydroxyl radicals, it is called a polyhydroxy alcohol. Ethyl alcohol is found in whisky, wines, and perfumes.

If the hydrogen atom is replaced by a CHO radical, which is called an aldehyde group, an aldehyde is formed (e.g., CH_3CHO-ethyl aldehyde). These are found in sugars, wheat, rice, and other carbohydrates.

If a CO radical, a ketone group, replaces the hydrogen, the resulting compound is ketone. An example of a ketone is acetone, which is found in nail polish.

If a COOH radical, an acid group, replaces the hydrogen, the resulting compound is a fatty acid. We talk of fats in the diet and fat related to body weight. Fatty acid is a type of fat that is found in our diets and in our bodies.

Bonds between Atoms

Two or more elements combine to form compounds. The elements combine with one another through links, also called bonds, to form stable compounds. If the bond between two carbon atoms in a fatty acid is single, the compound is called a saturated compound or a saturated fatty acid. However, if there are two or more bonds between the carbon atoms the resulting compound is called an unsaturated compound or unsaturated fatty acid. This is more important and relevant with respect to fats and fatty acids. A fatty acid with one double bond is called a monounsaturated fatty acid, and a fatty acid with multiple double bonds is called a polyunsaturated fatty acid. The saturated fats found in butter and cheese are unhealthy and predispose people to heart attacks, stroke, and hypertension. Olive oil, canola oil, and other vegetable oils have higher amounts of unsaturated fatty acids and are healthier.

A compound with ten carbon atoms is often referred to as a 10-C compound, one with twelve carbon atoms as a 12-C compound, and so on.

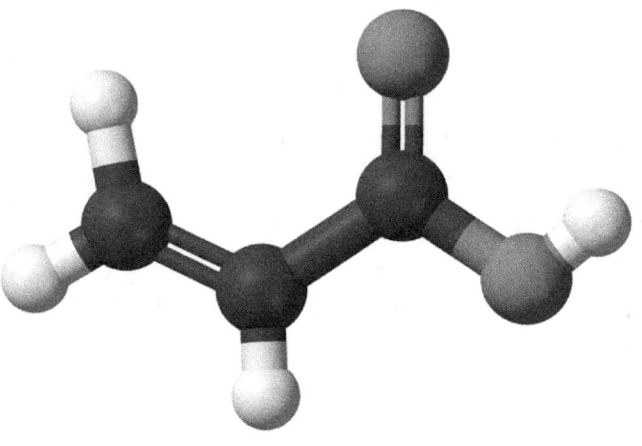

Propenoic acid, an unsaturated acid[29]

Now that we know something about hydrocarbons, let us discuss the three major constituents of food: carbohydrates, proteins, and fats, which are all hydrocarbons.

Carbohydrates

Carbohydrates are polyhydroxy alcohols with aldehyde or ketone groups. Carbohydrates are simple or complex. Simple carbohydrates are often referred to as sugars (e.g., naturally occurring sugars found in honey, milk, fruits, bread, and table sugar). Simple sugars, which are made of single units of six-carbon compounds, are called monosaccharides. Examples of monosaccharides are the glucose found in honey and the fructose found in fruits.

Sugar found in human blood is glucose, which is the primary source of energy for cells. Simple sugars with two six-carbon units combine to form disaccharides. Examples of disaccharides are maltose found in malt, lactose found in milk, sucrose in sugarcane, and table sugar. In the following paragraphs, blood glucose is often referred to as blood sugar.

Polysaccharides are complex sugars. An example is glycogen, which is a polymer of glucose and is found in liver and muscle cells. Glycogen is the storage form of glucose. Complex carbohydrates also form an important structural component of cells (such as the cell membrane).

A simple classification of carbohydrates is given in the table below.

Table 4.1: Types of Carbohydrates

Types of carbohydrates	Examples
Monosaccharides (one molecule of monosaccharide)	Glucose Fructose Galactose

Disaccharides (two molecules of monosaccharide)	Sucrose Maltose Lactose
Polysaccharides (many molecules of monosaccharide)	Starch Glycogen Cellulose

Glucose

This is a naturally occurring sugar in honey. It causes a fast and high rise in blood glucose levels when ingested. All carbohydrates break down mostly into monosaccharides during digestion in the intestine before their absorption. They are the main fuel from which the body derives energy.

Fructose

This commonly occurring natural sugar is present in fruits and honey. It does not cause a high rise in blood sugar levels when ingested. It is sweeter than cane sugar. Honey is a natural syrup that contains about 35 percent glucose and about 40 percent fructose.

Lactose

This is made of one molecule each of glucose and galactose linked together. It is the sugar present in milk. It is less sweet than cane sugar.

Maltose

This is made of two molecules of glucose linked together. It is less sweet than cane sugar.

Sucrose

This is cane sugar, and it is made of one molecule each of glucose and fructose. It is naturally present in sugarcane and sugar beets.

How are Simple and Complex Carbohydrates Relevant to Diabetes?

The simple carbohydrates, such as monosaccharides and disaccharides, are digested easily and quickly. They are rapidly absorbed from the intestine into the blood, resulting in a quick and high rise in blood sugar levels. This is not good in a diabetic, because the patient is unable to handle a heavy load of glucose as quickly as a healthy person. Moreover, high levels of blood sugar persist for longer periods in diabetics. Hence it is advisable for a diabetic not to eat foods that are rich in simple sugars, such as cane sugar, mangoes, and candy—at least not in high quantities.

Complex carbohydrates, in contrast, are digested and absorbed over longer periods and are therefore better suited for diabetic patients. The complex sugars are present in whole-wheat grains, oats, barley, and lentils.

Glycogen

This is a polymer of glucose. Several glucose units join to form a large molecule of glycogen.

Glycemic Index (GI)

Some years ago it was realized that different carbohydrates raise blood sugar levels to different degrees, although the calorie value is the same. The extent to which the level of blood glucose increases when one eats a particular food item is called its glycemic index (GI). The GI uses white bread, which is given the value of one hundred, as the baseline. If another food item of the same caloric value raises the blood glucose level to half the level of white bread on ingestion, the GI of that substance is 50.

Honey has a lower GI as compared to cane sugar, so if you must eat sugar, eat honey. Certain food items, such as whole-grain bread; unrefined cereals, such as oats; pasta; basmati rice; legumes; and lentils have low GIs in comparison to white bread, cornflakes, cakes, cookies, muffins, and ice cream. Fruits such as grapes, mangoes, and bananas have higher GIs as compared to apples, plums, guavas, papayas, and cantaloupes. Diabetic patients should consume food items with lower glycemic indexes.

Table 4.2: Glycemic Index of Common Foods[30]

Raisins	64
Cake	67
Croissants	67
Soft drinks	68
Mars bars	68
Muffins	69
Potatoes, mashed	70
Bagels	72

Popcorn	72
French fries	73
Donuts	76
Waffles	76
Table sugar	65
Pineapples	66
Bananas	53
Mangoes	55
Apples	36
Pears	36
Grapes	43
Oranges	43
Plums	24
Grapefruit	25
Peaches	28
Tomatoes	38
Yogurt	14
Milk, skim	32
Soybeans	18
Split peas	33
Lentils	29

Tortillas	38
Honey	73
Wheat bread	69
Rice, instant	87
Pizza, cheese	60
Mixed grains	45
Pasta	45

Proteins

Proteins are organic compounds. The building blocks of proteins are amino acids, which are radicals that contain nitrogen. There are several types of amino acids. Some can be produced in the body by other organic substances while others cannot. Those that can be synthesized by the body are called nonessential amino acids while those that need to be consumed in food are called essential amino acids.

Proteins constitute an innate portion of the structure and composition of the body. They form the muscles and are an integral component of all the cells.

Hormones, enzymes, and antibodies are some of the common protein molecules:

- Hormones control many functions. For example, the sex hormones are responsible for all sexual activity, including production of ova in females and sperm in males. Insulin, a hormone secreted by the pancreas, controls the metabolism of glucose.

- Enzymes in the digestive juices in the stomach and the intestine help in the digestion of food.
- Antibodies are substances secreted by the cells of the immune system to fight germs that may invade the body and cause disease.
- Proteins are critical for the health, structure, and function of the body.

Fats, or Lipids

If you put a drop of oil in water, it will not mix with the water. This is the defining property of fats, which are defined as substances not soluble in water but soluble in organic solvents, such as chloroform, benzene, xylene, etc. Common fats include fatty acids, triglycerides (compounds of glycerol, a base, and fatty acids), and cholesterol.

Fatty Acids

Fatty acids are compounds that contain COOH radicals. They are present in cooking oils. If you study the label on cooking fats, you may see words like *linolenic acid* or *stearic acid*—these are types of fatty acids. The fatty acids have variable lengths and numbers of carbon atoms; they may have sixteen or eighteen carbon atoms or be even longer chain carbon compounds. Cells also use fatty acids as fuel to obtain energy. When a person starves and glycogen stores are depleted, the person uses fats for energy requirements.

Triglycerides

Another type of fat, triglycerides are found in nature and are made of fatty acids and glycerol, commonly called glycerin (the substance often used to make ice cream).

Cholesterol

Cholesterol, another fat, is a complex compound found widely in nature. It is present in the yellow yolks of eggs. It is an important raw material used by the body in the synthesis of products such as steroids and sex hormones.

Because fats are not soluble in water, they cannot be transported in their native form in the blood, as blood is a water-based fluid. To enable fats to be carried in the circulation, a protein layer is required to coat them, making them water soluble. These complexes are called lipoproteins, which are tiny packets with envelopes made of protein, and the contents are fats such as cholesterol, triglycerides, and fatty acids. Cholesterol is a heavy and dense molecule. Hence packets that contain cholesterol are heavier and denser than those containing other types of fats. These are the high-density lipoproteins (HDL). Packets that contain more triglycerides and less cholesterol are lighter and are called low-density lipoproteins (LDL).

On the basis of their weight and density, lipoproteins are classified into high-density lipoproteins (HDL), low-density lipoproteins (LDL), very low-density lipoproteins (VLDL), and chylomicrons. HDL is a small, dense molecule while LDL is bigger and lighter than HDL. VLDL is still bigger and lighter, and chylomicrons are the lightest and the largest. As cholesterol is denser compared to triglycerides, there is more cholesterol in HDL and less in LDL and VLDL, and there are more triglycerides in chylomicrons as compared to other lipoproteins.

Table 4.3: Composition of Lipoproteins in Human Plasma

Fraction	Total lipids (percent)
Chylomicrons	98–99
VLDL	90–93
LDL	79
HDL	67

The table above shows the percentages of lipids in various lipo-proteins. The rest of the content is made up of proteins (e.g., chy-lomicrons are 98 to 99 percent fats and 1 to 2 percent proteins).

Digestion, Absorption, and the Storage of Fats

Fats taken in from meals are digested in the intestine and absorbed. They are transported in the circulation as chylomi-crons and later carried to the liver. They are rapidly metabo-lized in the liver and converted to other types of fats, such as HDL and LDL, which are then returned to the circulation.

Fats stored in fat depots such as subcutaneous tissue inside the abdomen—in the mesentery and omentum, which are folds of peritoneum, the lining of abdominal cavity—are mostly triglyc-erides. LDLs are considered harmful to the body, as high levels of LDL in the blood have been associated with increased risk of heart attack and stroke. Being a bigger and lighter molecule, LDL gets trapped in the vessel wall, causing arteriosclerosis, a disease of the blood vessels in which the arteries become rigid and thick, which is associated with a high risk of heart attack and stroke. The opposite holds true with HDL.

In times of need, such as during starvation, triglycerides from the fat depots are taken to the liver and broken down into fatty acids and glycerol. The fatty acids are further broken down into short-chain compounds called ketones. The ketones are transported in the circulation and carried to the cells, where they are burned to produce energy. This happens when the carbohydrates consumed do not fulfill the energy requirements of the body. This also happens in a diabetic when, due to lack of insulin, glucose cannot be used, and the patient depends on fats to fulfill the energy requirements. Since more triglycerides need to be transported in the circulation in people with uncontrolled diabetes, the level of triglycerides (and hence LDL cholesterol) is high in diabetics.

In people with type 1 diabetes, where insulin is lacking, the body heavily depends on ketones for its energy needs, often resulting in ketosis (high levels of ketones in the blood) and ketonuria (when level of ketones in the blood rises and ketones spill or overflow into urine).

It is important to know that nerve cells in the brain and spinal cord largely depend on glucose for their energy requirements.

Whenever the blood glucose level exceeds 180 mg percent, glucose starts getting excreted into the urine, as the renal threshold for glucose is 180 mg percent.

Table 4.4: Normal and Abnormal Levels of Fats in the Blood

Total blood cholesterol	
Normal	100–180 mg percent
High	>240 mg percent
HDL cholesterol	
Normal	35mg percent or higher
LDL cholesterol	
Normal	<130 mg percent or lower
Triglycerides	
Normal	150–200 mg percent or lower
Total lipids	
Normal range	400–1,000 mg percent

It is recommended that LDL levels should not exceed 100 mg percent. This is especially for those who have high risk of heart attacks, such as diabetics.[31]

CHAPTER 5

Normal Body Functions

It is crucial to imbibe the normal so as to understand the abnormal.
—Rita Malik

This chapter is devoted to the normal functioning of the human system. It does not give the intricate details but skims the surface.

The human body is made of millions of cells. Cells are like tiny bricks, akin to building blocks in LEGO sets, that assemble to form the various systems. Cells are of several types and collect to form organs and structures (tissues) such as the heart, lungs, liver, and muscles. The cells perform specialized functions.

Human physiology details how the cells derive energy from the food we eat and how they perform the myriad functions that sustain life.

The food we eat gives energy to the cells to execute mechanical, chemical, and electrical activities. The mechanical functions include physical activities such as running, walking, eating, talking, etc. The chemical functions include the synthesis of digestive juices, the formation of hormones (such as sex hormones for sexual activity), the secretion of growth hormone, and many more. The electrical impulses generated in nerve cells in the brain and spinal cord are transmitted through the nerves. For example, when the brain commands the leg muscles to run, the signal travels along the nerves, which conduct the electrical impulse from the brain to the legs.

Cells need energy to perform their various functions. Each cell absorbs glucose and oxygen from the blood, and within the cell, glucose is broken down to release energy. The oxygen present in circulating blood enters the cells and burns glucose to release energy.

The three main constituents of food—carbohydrates, fats, and proteins—are used as the burning fuel to provide energy. Carbohydrate is by far the most important source of energy. The body undertakes a network of reactions to achieve this end. When carbohydrates are broken down, glucose is released. It is the principal substance involved in the intricate set of chemical reactions to liberate energy.[32]

Table 5.1: Approximate Calories of Three Main Foods

Food type (1 g)	Energy contents
Carbohydrates	4 calories
Fats	9 calories
Proteins	4 calories

Digestion of the Food We Eat

We chew food with the help of saliva. It trickles down the food pipe, which is in the middle of the chest, behind the windpipe. From the food pipe, food enters the stomach, which lies beneath the diaphragm (a muscular partition that separates the chest from the abdomen). The trunk of the body is divided into two compartments: the upper chest and the lower abdomen.

The food is mixed in the stomach with gastric juice. It is churned to form a thin gruel over a period of about three hours. It is then gradually squeezed into the first part of the intestines (gut). Bile is a green fluid that is formed in the liver and stored in the gallbladder. Bile and digestive juices from the pancreas pour through a duct into this portion of the intestines. The gruel is further changed into a thin fluid, and the food constituents are broken into simple compounds. In the course of diges-

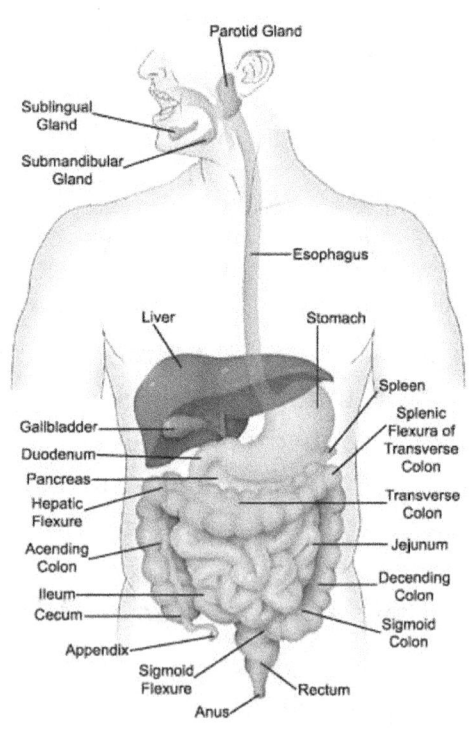

View of the chest and abdomen.[34]

tion, all carbohydrates, including starch, are changed into monosaccharides or disaccharides. The monosaccharides are mostly glucose and fructose, a simple sugar found in fruits. The fats are split into fatty acids and glycerol, and the proteins are split into amino acids.[33]

Organs of the chest, abdomen, and pelvis are depicted here:

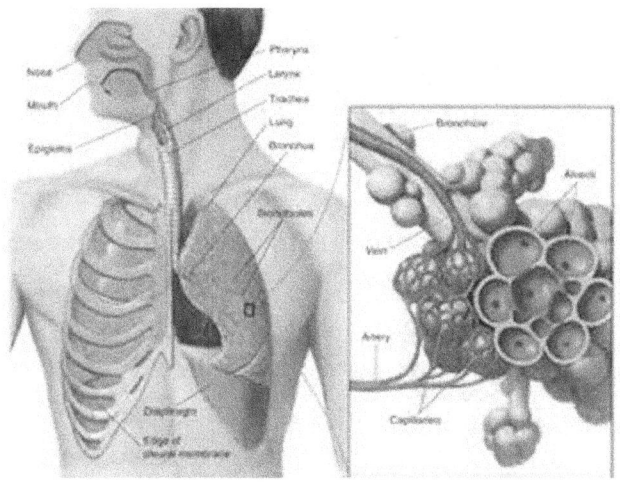

Respiratory system—Jessica and Ayako respiratory system[35]

Absorption of Food

These simple molecules (compounds) are slowly absorbed from the intestinal tract and enter the bloodstream. The particles are taken to the liver by the bloodstream. The liver is the main workshop that handles food constituents.

The liver can also form glucose from the food constituents brought to it by the blood from the intestines by splitting or by conversion. For example, it can convert fructose into glucose. Glucose, thus created, reenters the blood from the liver, where it is picked up by the cells. Moving glucose into the cells is a complex function. Insulin, a hormone secreted by the pancreas, facilitates the passage of glucose into the cells, where it is burned to release energy. An optimum glucose level in the blood is necessary to keep the cells from starving, and the liver and insulin maintain a constant level of glucose, so the body is never deprived of its essential fuel. Whenever the glucose levels fall due to starvation or excessive use, the liver rapidly goes into action, synthesizes more glucose, and pours it into the blood. Whenever the level of glucose rises, the pancreas secretes insulin, which helps shift glucose into the liver and muscles, where it can be stored as glycogen.

The body also derives energy from fatty acids that are obtained from the fats we eat. However, the nerve cells in the brain and spinal cord almost exclusively depend on glucose for their functional requirements. Anytime blood glucose levels fall below a critical value, a person may feel dizzy or faint. A blood glucose level of about 80 to 140 mg percent is crucial for healthy functioning. Whenever blood glucose levels change, sensors all over the body get alerted, and signals flow to and fro to restore the levels. Insulin plays a vital role.

Excess glucose that enters the bloodstream after ingestion of food is converted into glycogen in the liver with the help of insulin. Glycogen is formed as glucose molecules strung together. When the glucose in the blood is depleted, glycogen in the liver is changed back into glucose and thrown into the bloodstream.

Carbohydrates eaten in excess of the body's energy requirement are changed into fat, which is the body's energy store. Glycogen is the short-term storage form of food, and fat is the long-term storage form. In times of starvation, the body calls on fat stores to fulfill its needs.

Maintenance of the Interior Milieu

Claude Bernard, a renowned physician born in France (1813–1878), stated that the internal milieu (the internal composition of body) must be kept in a steady state, and it is imperative for the viability of the cells that the internal environment is maintained in a steady state. The body is endowed with a mechanism to do so. For instance, in cold weather the metabolic rate goes up, and heat is generated to maintain body temperature. The reverse happens in warm weather. Whether it is body temperature, blood oxygen, or blood glucose levels, any shift in the normal range triggers a set of reactions, and the body makes the necessary adjustments. This restores the internal environment to its original state.

CHAPTER 6

Insulin and Its Mode of Action

Facts Not Fiction

In earlier chapters we explored the major constituents of food, how the food we eat is digested and absorbed from the intestine, how it is taken to the liver and changed into glucose, and how it is passed into the circulatory system, making it available to the cells for their energy requirements.

Insulin plays a pivotal role in health and well-being. It plays a key role in how the body uses sugars. This chapter explains insulin's mode of action, the maintenance of blood glucose levels, and the regulation of insulin secretion.[36]

Diabetes is a disease wherein the glucose metabolism is deranged. In order to understand diabetes, it is essential to understand the action of insulin, which controls the passage or entry of glucose into the cells. As an analogy, the cell has a door with a handle that has to be unlocked and turned. Insulin fits like a key into the lock, turns the handle, and opens the door so glucose can enter the cell.

Insulin

The discovery of insulin was a revolution that laid the foundation for the understanding, treatment, and prevention of diabetes.

The pancreas is unique as it performs both endocrine and exocrine functions. It secretes insulin, which enters the bloodstream directly (the endocrine function) and secretes digestive juices, which enter the intestine through ducts (the exocrine function).

A gland is an organ that makes substances; for example, the mammary glands make milk, and the sweat glands secrete sweat. Glands that pour secretions into ducts are called *exocrine glands* while glands that pour secretions into the bloodstream are called endocrine glands.

The pancreas is a large endocrine gland in the upper part of the abdomen, behind the stomach. It has a head, a body, and a tail. Scattered throughout the pancreas are clusters of cells called the islets of Langerhans (named after German pathologist Paul Langerhans, who first described the cells). The pancreas has more than a million clusters of these islets. There are more islets located in the tail of the pancreas as compared to the body and the head. Within these islets are cells called beta (β) cells, which form and store insulin.

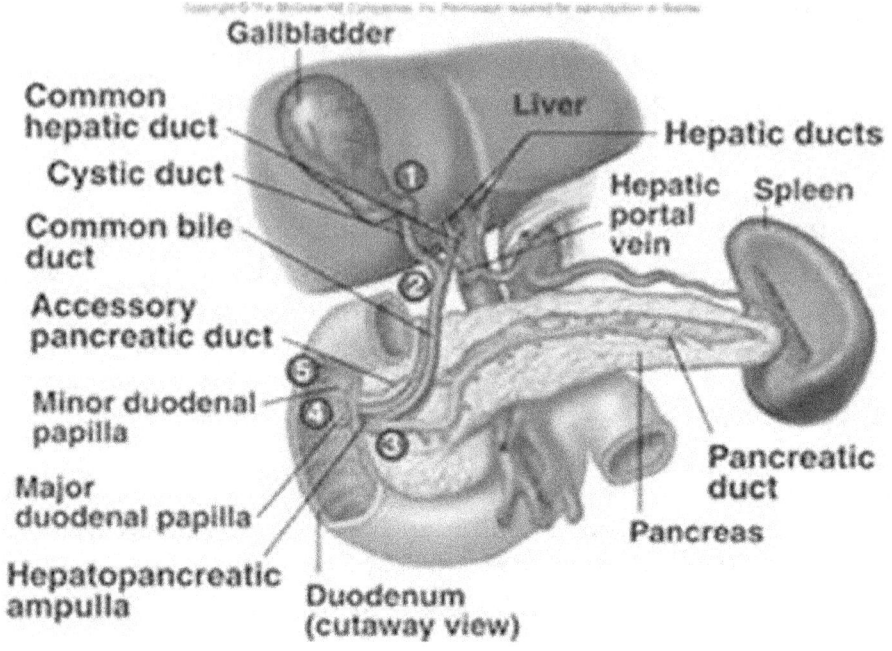

Gallbladder

Common
hepatic duct

Cystic duct

Common bile
duct

Accessory
pancreatic duct

Minor duodenal
papilla

Major
duodenal papilla

Hepatopancreatic
ampulla

Liver

Hepatic ducts

Hepatic
portal
vein

Spleen

Pancreatic
duct

Pancreas

Duodenum
(cutaway view)

The pancreas and spleen[37]

The Mechanism of Insulin Secretion

The formation and secretion of insulin is directly proportional to the level of glucose in the blood in healthy persons. This is a finely tuned and monitored mechanism that maintains the optimum level of glucose.[38] Whenever the blood glucose level rises, insulin is secreted and helps bring down the glucose level. Whenever the blood level of glucose falls, insulin is withdrawn from the circulation. When the level of glucose rises, insulin brings it down. This is achieved in two ways: by transferring glucose from the blood into the body cells and by converting glucose into glycogen within the liver cells and the skeletal muscle (voluntary muscles) cells. Insulin binds to receptors present on tissue cells, which facilitates the entry of glucose into the cells. These receptors are like locks into which insulin fits like a key, and it opens the door through which glucose gains entry into the cell. An exception occurs in the brain cells and red blood cells, which imbibe glucose without the help of receptors. In the liver the glycogen store is a reserve that the body calls on in time of need.

After a meal food is digested in the intestine, and a large amount of glucose is absorbed into the blood. This extra amount of glucose is stored in the liver in the form of glycogen, and when needed it is changed back into glucose and used to fulfill energy requirements. Whenever the blood glucose level falls, the secretion of insulin by the pancreas is withdrawn. However, when blood glucose falls to dangerously low levels (called hypoglycemia), other hormones come into action. These hormones include adrenaline, secreted by the adrenal glands in the abdomen; and growth factor 1, secreted by the pituitary gland at the base of brain. They change glycogen in the liver into glucose and throw it into the bloodstream, where the cells can pick it up. The glycogen store in the muscle cells is broken into glucose and used during physical activity.

Normally the islets of Langerhans maintain a perfect balance and monitor blood glucose levels by releasing appropriate amounts of insulin. In a person with diabetes, this balance breaks down.

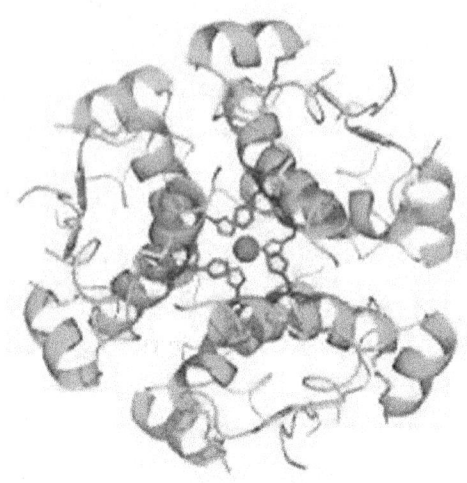

The Structure of Insulin Molecule[39]

The figure below summarizes insulin's actions. The activated insulin receptor speeds the uptake of amino acids and glucose and activates protein synthesis from amino acids and glycogen and triglyceride synthesis from glucose. Insulin inhibits the breakdown of triglycerides in adipose tissue and gluconeogenesis (the formation of glucose from other food ingredients) in the liver.

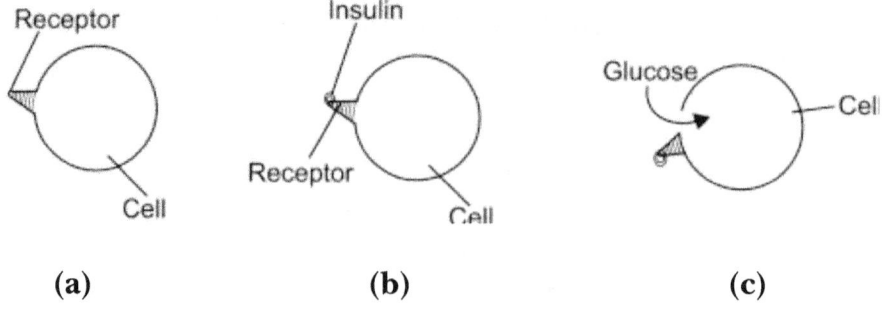

Diagrammatic representation of the action of insulin

(a) Shows a cell with a receptor.

(b) Shows insulin linked to the cell receptor.

(c) The link between insulin and the receptor facilitates glucose entry into the cell; a defect in the link causes insulin resistance.

The Role of Glucagon in Glucose Level Maintenance

Besides beta (β) cells, there are alpha (α) cells in the islets of Langerhans. The alpha cells secrete a hormone called glucagon, and it plays a role opposite to that of insulin: it tends to increase blood glucose levels. It does so by stimulating the liver to change glycogen into glucose and throw it into the bloodstream. It comes into action in hypoglycemia along with adrenaline. It also helps maintain the normal equilibrium of blood glucose along with insulin and the liver.

By releasing calibrated amounts of insulin and glucagon, the pancreas masterminds healthy blood glucose levels and prevents dramatic swings in blood sugar levels. Besides regulating metabolism insulin promotes the growth and multiplication of cells.

Blood Sugar Regulation

Two hormones are responsible for controlling the concentration of glucose in the blood: insulin and glucagon.

The graphic below depicts the absorption of glucose from the gastrointestinal tract into the bloodstream; from there it is taken to the liver and muscles, where it is stored as glycogen. The muscles use glycogen for energy during exercise. The glycogen stores in the liver are available for the energy needs of the whole body.

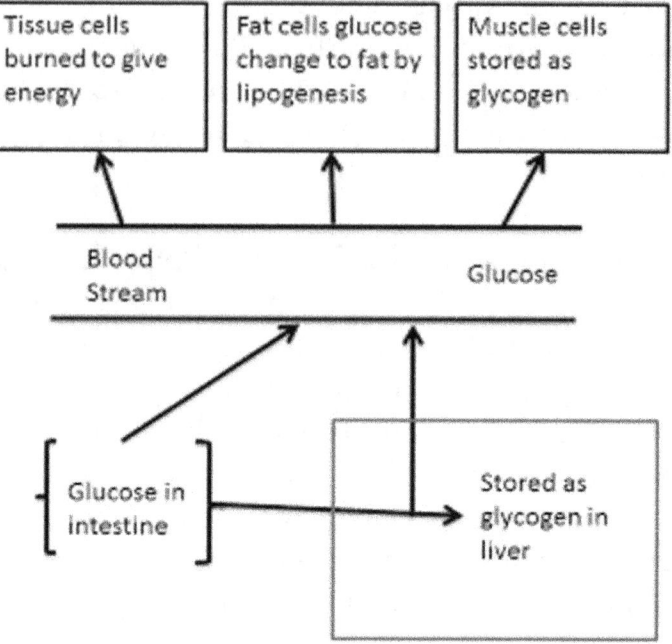

Diagrammatic representation of glucose circulation.

PART 2

CHAPTER 7

Symptoms of Diabetes

Monitor and observe any change in your body.

The awareness of diabetes is exceedingly low because most people are not familiar with its presenting features. This chapter describes the modes of presentation as well as its association with hypertension and obesity.

A long time ago, my husband and I were on holiday in Europe. My husband drank a lot of beer during the trip and, to my annoyance, went to the toilet frequently. I had to shell out money for the beer as well as his frequent visits to the toilet. At that time we did not realize what was happening. On our return home, we noticed he had lost lot of weight. We knew something had gone wrong and had his blood sugar tested. It turned out to be 600 mg percent—a very high level.

The symptoms of diabetes are often ignored for some time. People may feel hungry all the time and have an uncontrollable desire to eat. They may pass urine more often and get up several times during the night to urinate. Sometimes they have visual disturbances such as blurred or double vision. They may have severe pain radiating in their thighs or numbness or tingling in their feet.

These signs should never to be ignored:
1. Increased appetite.
2. Increased thirst.
3. Increased urination.
4. Unexplained loss of weight.
5. A nonhealing wound or ulcer.
6. Severe nerve pain.
7. Sudden visual disturbances.
8. High blood pressure.
9. High blood lipids.
10. Frequent eruptions of boils.

A yearly routine checkup including a blood profile at a primary health-care center will help individuals keep track of their lipid levels.

If any of these symptoms occur, the person should get his or her blood sugar tested.

Type 1 Diabetes

Type 1 diabetes is referred to as insulin-dependent diabetes. It usually occurs in people fewer than thirty years of age but may occur at any age. The symptoms often come on suddenly and severely. Patients present more dramatically than those with type 2 diabetes and have polyuria (increased frequency of urination), polydipsia (increased thirst), polyphagia (increased hunger), and weight loss.

Type 2 Diabetes

Patients with type 2 diabetes may or may not have the symptoms noted above, and they tend to have more obscure presentations. They may feel fatigue or tingling or numbness in the hands or feet, and they may experience blurred vision. A nonhealing wound or itching (e.g., vaginitis) may be the first sign. Hypertension (high blood pressure) or a heart attack may be the first sign of this serious disease.

Impaired Glucose Tolerance

IGT is a kind of prediabetic phase. The person is unable to handle glucose as effectively as a healthy individual. The fasting blood glucose level remains higher than in a healthy person but not as high as in someone with diabetes.

Non-Insulin-Dependent Diabetes and IGT

The physical and metabolic characteristics of people with non-insulin-dependent diabetes mellitus (NIDDM) and IGT have been analyzed in great detail. The data collected from the National Health Interview Survey (NHIS) in the United States shows that the mean body mass index (BMI) is highest in persons with NIDDM followed by those with IGT and then those with normal glucose tolerance.

Among people with NIDDM, the frequency of obesity is much higher in women (46.6 percent) than in men (20.9 percent). The incidence of obesity in women with type 2 diabetes is higher than in men. It has been noted that the tendency to be obese exists in those with a predisposition to diabetes as well as those with impaired glucose tolerance. The incidence of obesity is even higher in African-American women (69.5 percent).

Central (abdominal) obesity is more evident in persons with NIDDM and IGT as compared to healthy individuals. Mean blood pressure levels are also higher in persons with NIDDM and IGT as compared to healthy persons. Hypertension (blood pressure greater than 130/95 mm Hg) in persons age sixty-five to seventy-four affects 60 percent of those with NIDDM, 50.7 percent of those with IGT, and 38.3 percent of those with normal glucose tolerance.

Lipid Profile

A similar tendency is observed in the lipid profile (the levels of various types of lipids). The levels of total cholesterol, LDL cholesterol, and triglycerides are higher in persons with NIDDM and IGT as compared to persons with normal glucose tolerance. The level of HDL cholesterol, which is healthy cholesterol, is lower in persons with NIDDM and IGT and higher in individuals with normal glucose tolerance.

CHAPTER 8

Definitions and Classifications of Diabetes

Natural forces within us are the true healers of disease.
- Hippocrates

What are diabetes mellitus and its variants? What is the role of heredity? What is insulin resistance? What does it imply, and is there anything we can do about it? These subjects are touched upon in the following pages, as is the role of immunity.

The two major variants of diabetes are type 1 and type 2. The fundamental difference is that in type 1, there is a total or an almost total lack of insulin whereas in type 2 some amount of insulin is still available in the body.

Diabetes mellitus is characterized by hyperglycemia (high blood glucose levels due to a complete or relative deficiency of insulin or insensitivity of the tissues to circulating insulin). Due to the lack of insulin, the cells fail to metabolize (use) glucose, and as a result the glucose in the blood remains high.

Diabetes has three main characteristics:

1. The failure of glucose to pass from blood into cells, either due to a lack of insulin or insulin resistance (insulin attaches itself to receptors on the cell surface and facilitates the flow of glucose into the cell; a defect in insulin-receptor link hinders this function). A similar insulin resistance at the level of the brain fails to suppress appetite, causing obesity. To overcome insulin resistance the pancreas secretes more insulin. Pancreatic beta cells become exhausted and die of fatigue, resulting in beta cell failure and type 2 diabetes.

2. As discussed earlier, insulin unlocks the doors of cells, allowing glucose to flow into them. When insulin is lacking, this function is impaired. This is true in type 1 diabetes but not in all cases of type 2.

3. In type 2 diabetes, often the insulin key is unable to fit into the lock on the cell and open the door (insulin resistance). Even when an adequate amount of insulin is available, it is unable to operate because the key-and-lock mechanism is deranged. As a result glucose is unable to flow into the cells, and it remains high in the blood while the cells continue to starve.

Normal fasting blood glucose, which is measured after eight hours of fasting (as a routine, early in the morning) is less than 100 mg percent. A reading between 100 mg percent and 126 mg percent is considered IGT, and a level above 126 mg percent is diagnosed as diabetes. The blood glucose level measured two hours after a glucose load or a proper meal is less than 140 mg percent in normal cases, between 140 mg percent and 199 mg percent in persons with IGT, and greater than 200 mg percent in persons with diabetes. Blood glucose levels can be expressed in mg percent (i.e., milligrams per deciliter [mg/dL] of blood) and as millimoles per liter (mmol/L). To convert mg/dL into mmol/L, multiply the milligrams by 0.055. To convert mmol/L into mg/dL, multiply the millimoles by 18.01.

Table 8.1: Equivalents between mg/dL and mmol/l

50 mg/dL	2.8 mmol/L
100 mg/dL	5.6 mmol/L
150 mg/dL	8.3 mmol/L
200 mg/dL	11.1 mmol/L

Four major types of diabetes have been defined by the WHO and the National Diabetic Data Group (NDDG): insulin-dependent diabetes mellitus (IDDM), non-insulin-dependent diabetes mellitus (NIDDM), gestational diabetes mellitus (GDM), and others that are secondary to other diseases.

Type 1 Diabetes, Also Called IDDM

It is also known as juvenile diabetes. In this variant insulin is almost totally deficient.[41] It comprises 10 percent of all diabetes cases. It manifests in the juvenile age group but can occur at any age and is occasionally seen in nonobese adults. It usually becomes manifest before the age of thirty. The patient requires insulin from an external source because the pancreas is unable to produce insulin. There are genetic predispositions and environmental influences in the development of the disease.

Blood has red cells, which carry oxygen, and white cells, which help in the body's defense. Among the white blood cells are lymphocytes, further classified into B and T types. B lymphocytes form antibodies and T lymphocytes kill foreign cells as bacteria. Type 1 diabetes is an autoimmune disorder wherein the body's T lymphocytes destroy the b cells of the pancreas.

Immune Dysfunction in Type 1 Diabetes

The body is endowed with an immune or defense system. Like any military it has its range of weapons. The white cells in the blood are akin to guns, and the antibodies are akin to bullets. When a germ enters the body, the defense system manufactures antibodies to kill it. Antibodies are formed by B lymphocytes.

Antibodies are protein in nature. They are generated as part of the body's defense mechanism in response to antigens, which under normal circumstances are foreign proteins or protein complexes. In other words antibodies are like missiles that attack foreign invaders (antigens). They damage or inactivate the antigen against which they have been produced. For example, when bacteria (foreign invaders) infect a person, the body regards them as alien. As part of its complicated defense arsenal, it forms antibodies to inactivate the bacterial proteins, which are the antigens.

Normally the body does not form antibodies against its own cells, but sometimes this function goes haywire. In this variant of diabetes, an autoimmune disorder exists. The immune system starts manufacturing missiles (antibodies) against its own cells and destroys them. The patient develops antibodies against his or her own insulin and pancreatic beta islet cells.

It could also be possible that the pancreatic cell surface antigens, by which the immune system recognizes the cells as self, are altered and defy recognition. Every cell in the body has surface markers. These are a kind of ID by which the cells are recognized as self instead of as foreign cells, such as viruses. If the ID of the cell is damaged, the cell will be regarded as foreign and killed.

Thus in type 1 diabetes, there is an immune dysfunction. The immune system starts forming antibodies against its own pancreatic beta cells, which manufacture insulin. With the inactivation of these cells, the production of insulin is greatly reduced, and the patient is totally dependent on insulin from an external source.[42] Evidence in favor of the autoimmune mechanism in the development of type 1 diabetes is the presence of specific antibodies against pancreatic beta cells in the patient's blood.

Genetic Control of Type 1 Diabetes

Genes determine human characteristics and control the body's functions. There is a strong genetic predisposition to and association with HLA-DR3 or HLA-DR4 in type 1 diabetes. The human genome is a lengthy sequence of genes, and they have specific nomenclature. HLA-DR3 and HLA-DR4 are the genes that control the body's immune response and are associated with tissue matching and compatibility.

T lymphocytes are a class of white blood cells that play an important role in the regulation of the immune response. T lymphocytes are part of the body's vast arsenal that produces chemicals (among them antibodies) to fight foreign invaders and disease germs. The association of type 1 diabetes with the genetic code dealing with defense mechanisms indicates a strong link between heredity, immunity, and type 1 diabetes.

Often a viral infection, such as mumps or German measles, precipitates the autoimmune process.[43,44]

Ketosis and ketonuria (the presence of ketone bodies in blood and urine, respectively), both life-threatening conditions, can occur in this type of diabetes.

Another advance in this direction has been the discovery of TAP1 and TAP2 genes, which control the IDs of cells. These genes have been found to influence the interaction between cell surface antigens and the immune system.[45]

Type 2 Diabetes (NIDDM)

Although environmental factors such as a sedentary lifestyle play an important role in the genesis of type 2 diabetes, genetic factors are even more important. In the early stages of type 2 diabetes, the patient does not require an external source of insulin.

All characteristics of our bodies are hereditary, passing from parents to offspring by virtue of their genes, and genes control all the functions of the body. Some functions are controlled by single genes, while others are under the influences of several genes. If five genes control a process, a defect in any one of them will cause disease. Hence a disease may have several genetic causes.

Type 2 diabetes is an example. It is divided into several types based on genetic defects, and it forms a heterogeneous group. It is divided into obese and nonobese types.

Table 8.2: Differences between the Two Main Types of Diabetes

Type 1 diabetes	Type 2 diabetes
Age of onset: juvenile	Age of onset: adult
Intensity: severe	Intensity: less severe
Cause: heredity	Cause: obesity and heredity
Ketosis: usually present	Ketosis: usually absent
Ketonuria: usually present	Ketonuria: usually absent
Absolute dependence on insulin	May or may not require insulin

Insulin Resistance

In more than 90 percent of patients with type 2 diabetes, there is evidence of insulin resistance.[46,47,48,49] The tissues of the body, especially the liver, muscles, and fat, require extra insulin to maintain normal glycemic control as compared to healthy persons. As the tissues fail to respond to the normal levels of insulin and fail to use the glucose present in the blood, the level of glucose rises. In response the pancreas increases insulin. Insulin resistance in the periphery results in increased production of insulin by the pancreas, and this result in high levels of insulin in the blood.

Insulin resistance can occur even before diabetes becomes manifest. In the early phases, the pancreas secretes extra insulin to compensate for this resistance, so blood glucose levels remain within normal limits. Later the pancreas fails to keep up with the extra demand. As the blood glucose goes up, type 2 diabetes becomes manifest.

It is now believed that any degree of insulin resistance increases a person's risk of heart disease. Insulin resistance is associated with inflammatory cytokines and cardiovascular disease.[50,51] Drugs like Actos and Avandia act primarily by making muscle and fat tissues more responsive to insulin. They use glucose more effectively and readily and thereby bring down blood glucose levels. Targretin, a drug on trial, has been found to lower insulin resistance.

Insulin resistance is predominantly found in adults over the age of forty,[52] but it can occur in younger individuals, especially in Native Americans.

Insulin Resistance in Type 2 Diabetes

NIDDM often involves insulin resistance. Two defects characterize this disease: the failure of the tissue cells to respond to insulin and the failure of the pancreatic cells to produce adequate amounts of insulin in the face of hyperglycemia. As the cells fail to respond to insulin, the beta cells of the pancreas produce more insulin to overcome the resistance. At this stage the level of insulin in the blood is higher than normal, although it is ineffective. However, after some time the pancreatic cells become exhausted and begin to fail. With beta cell failure, the level of insulin starts to fall.[53]

This main form of NIDDM, associated with insulin resistance and beta cell failure, may comprise several etiologic (causative) entities that are both genetic and nongenetic. Many rare genetic syndromes are associated with glucose intolerance. Both insulin resistance (failure of insulin action to transport glucose from the circulation into the cells) and beta cell failure (lack of production of adequate amounts of insulin) have multiple genetic causes and result in many types of NIDDM. Beta cell failure may be secondary to insulin resistance, which may be concurrent with or even precede it. It is estimated that 50 percent of beta cell dysfunction is present at the time of diagnosis and increases with time.

Diabetes has strong familial and genetic predispositions. In identical twins, if one twin develops diabetes, the other will also have it. Type 2 diabetes is further divided into obese and non-obese variants.

Obesity: Insulin-Resistant Type 2 Diabetes

In this class of diabetes, the cells of the body tissues show decreased response to insulin present in the circulation. Even when adequate amounts of insulin are available, the cells fail to respond to it and do not get enough glucose for their energy needs. The cells starve even when the levels of glucose in the blood are high. The pancreas also reveals a decreased responsiveness to variations in the glucose levels in the blood. Even when the level of glucose is high, with beta cell failure the pancreas fails to secrete insulin to bring the level down.

Visceral obesity (an excessive amount of fat inside the abdomen) causes insulin resistance.[54,55]

PC1 Protein

This compound is more prevalent in people with type 2 diabetics than in nondiabetics. The overproduction of this substance is genetically determined. It is believed to interfere with the normal functioning of insulin receptors.

Type 1 Diabetes Is More Severe than Type 2

Type 2 differs from type 1 in that ketosis and ketonuria usually do not occur. This variant is also not linked to HLA genes, nor is there any autoimmune reaction. However, type 2 is more common than type 1, and 90 percent of diabetic patients have type 2.

Both types are complex diseases that arise from defective genes. A number of genes are involved in the formation, secretion, and use of insulin, and any subtle variation in the gene results in a defective gene. These abnormal genes interact with other genes and the environment. In type 1 diabetes, the susceptible gene reacts to environmental triggers, such as viruses. In type 2 diabetes, the genes react to external influences like obesity and inactivity, resulting in the development of diabetes or a greater risk of getting the disease.

Genetic Research in Diabetes

The International Type 2 Diabetes Genetic Linkage Consortium was formed to help researchers combine their individual findings, localize various genes, and determine their modes of function.[56] Once the genes are localized, it will help scientists develop drugs that target these genes and strategies to cure and prevent diabetes.

Dr. Graenne Bell and Dr. Nancy Cox of the University of Chicago have identified a gene called NIDDM1 on chromosome 2, which interacts with a gene on chromosome 15, resulting in an increased risk of developing type 2 diabetes. A defective NIDDM1 has been identified in two North European and

Mexican American population groups. Five maturity-onset diabetes of the young (MODY) genes[57] have also been identified. Another defective gene, which predisposes the Pima Indians to early kidney failure, has been localized. Pima Indians are a tribe who lived in that part of the United States that now is central and southern Arizona.

Research in the field of cell signaling, communication, and regulation by means of cytokines (specific molecules) has helped scientists understand the working of the immune system and what goes wrong in disorders such as type 1 diabetes. This is also shedding light on insulin resistance, which precedes type 2 diabetes.

Nuclear Hormone Receptors Regulate Gene Expressions

Receptors are structures on the cell surfaces. They link to other molecules and set in motion a cycle of reactions. For example, certain brain receptors link to insulin and set a cycle in motion that suppresses appetite. When these receptors are absent or defective, appetite is not suppressed, and a person has tendency to eat more and become obese.

This shows that a complex network of molecular signals and feedback loops involving the brain and other tissues are the keys to unraveling the mystery of the obesity and insulin resistance that precede type 2 diabetes.[58]

Besides these two main types, there some less common forms of diabetes.

Gestational Diabetes Mellitus (GDM)

This type of diabetes develops during pregnancy. The incidence among pregnant women is about 3 to 5 percent. Such subjects revert to normal when pregnancy ends, but 35 to 50 percent of such women progress to non-insulin-dependent diabetes later in life, especially if they are overweight. GDM is also associated with obesity, positive family history, and older age. Investigators believe the same genetic defects are present in these individuals as in those with type 2 diabetes.[59]

The prevalence of congenital birth defects in infants born to diabetic mothers is about 10 percent. About 3 to 5 percent of pregnancies in diabetic women result in the deaths of the newborns. Premature births, complications at delivery, and risks to the infants can develop.

This variant may remain asymptomatic, or the patient may develop symptoms similar to other types of diabetes. A regular blood sugar test is imperative, especially in high-risk women.

The cause of this variant is not fully understood. Some scientists believe that unrecognized diabetes is already present in such cases, and weight gain and hormonal alterations precipitate and unmask the disease.

Others Forms of Diabetes (Secondary Diabetes)

The prevalence of other variants is 1 to 2 percent of the total incidence of the disease.

Beta cell mass in the pancreas is reduced in certain conditions (e.g., in malignant disease of the pancreas and surgical removal of the pancreas). When pancreatitis (an inflammatory disease of the pancreas) develops, the functional beta cell mass is destroyed.

Pancreatitis is common in South India. Secondary diabetes is common in children due to severe protein malnutrition in third world countries like India, Indonesia, and Jamaica.

In some cases of secondary diabetes, there is a relative deficiency of insulin due to the overproduction of a group of hormones that are antagonistic to insulin.

Besides the three major forms of diabetes, other less significant variants exist. Their significances lie in the fact that they may lead to misdiagnoses of diabetes.

Some other causes of secondary diabetes include the following:
1. Chemical agents toxic to the beta cells of the pancreas, such as pentamidine and vacor, that reduce the beta cell mass
2. Genetic defects in -cell function
3. MODY 1, 2, 3, 4, 5
4. Genetic defects in insulin function.
5. Exocrine pancreatic diseases (e.g., pancreatitis, carcinoma, and cystic fibrosis)
6. Other endocrinopathies (see table 9.2)
7. Drugs or chemicals
8. Infections (e.g., congenital rubella and cytomegalovirus)
9. Drugs that increase blood sugar levels:
   Chlorthalidone
   Diazoxide
   Furosemide
   Epinephrine

Estrogen
Nicotinic acid
Phenytoin
Thyroid preparations
Thiazide
Glucagon
Caffeine
Morphine

10. Drugs that lower blood sugar levels:
Alcohol
Insulin
Beta-blockers
Anabolic steroids
Fenfluramine
Salicylates
Phenobarbital

Those drugs that raise blood sugar levels mimic diabetes and, along with other secondary causes of hyperglycemia, should be taken into consideration in the diagnosis of diabetes.

CHAPTER 9

Diagnosing Diabetes

Hard Talk

How can you know that you have diabetes and be sure it is not something else? This chapter discusses WHO diagnostic criteria, how to monitor blood sugar levels, the significance of urine examination, and when and why to do these tests. Other conditions associated with high blood glucose levels are also tabulated.

Laboratory Tests for the Diagnosis of Diabetes

In a person suspected to be suffering from diabetes, a diagnosis can be established by blood tests and urine analysis.

A simple, specific, and convenient test to detect the presence of glucose in urine can be done with the help of paper strips marketed as Diastix. These help detect as little as 0.1 percent of glucose in the urine. The color change in the strip gives a rough estimate of the amount of glucose present in the urine. However, certain drugs, especially if taken in large doses, such as aspirin and vitamin C, can interfere with the test results. A urine test is not advocated for the diagnosis of diabetes or recommended for day-to-day management. Laboratory tests for detection of ketone bodies in the urine are accepted, and in type 1 diabetes they are performed routinely.

Blood Glucose Test

The criterion for confirming diabetes is the estimation of blood glucose levels. A fasting plasma glucose level of 100 mg percent or more on more than one occasion helps establish the diagnosis. A normal fasting glucose level is up to 100 mg percent. If the fasting plasma glucose level is borderline, a standardized oral glucose tolerance test may be done, keeping the age factor in mind.

IGT is a class that encompasses persons whose glucose tolerances are between a healthy person's and a diabetic patient's. They constitute about 11 percent of adults, and these patients have higher risks of developing frank diabetes. Their fasting glucose levels are between 100 and 126 mg percent.

An international expert committee, sponsored by the ADA, recently made recommendations for the diagnosis, screening, and testing for diabetes mellitus.[60] Fasting plasma glucose is the preferred test for diagnosis and screening. The committee recommends it over oral glucose tolerance because it is reproducible, cost effective, and easier to perform.

Glycosylated Hemoglobin (HbA1c) Measurement

Glucose molecules in the blood combine with hemoglobin in red blood cells to form a stable compound called glycosylated hemoglobin (HbA1c). The higher the level of glucose in the blood, the higher the amount of HbA1c formed. In diabetics, because levels of glucose are higher than normal, the HbA1c estimates are also higher than normal. The life of red blood cells is three months on average, and these values of HbA1c persist for three months. If the estimated level of HbA1c is more than normal, it indicates that the glucose level has remained high for the previous three months. These estimates reflect the level of metabolic control over the previous three-month period. Such evaluations are important in the control and management of diabetes. The results of the Diabetes Control Complications Trial (DCCT) showed a direct relationship between HbA1c values and the risk of developing chronic complications.[61,62,63]

Fructosamine Assay

Another test available is the assay of fructosamine. It reflects the glycemic control over the previous one to two weeks. Fructosamine is a compound formed by the combination of fructose with amine. Its assay reflects the level of blood sugar in the previous two to three weeks. It has limited clinical value.[64]

These two tests, HbA1c and fructosamine level estimation, are a useful complement to the daily monitoring of blood glucose in achieving optimal glucose control, and they should not be used as a substitute for the latter. These tests (HbA1c and fructosamine assay) are not recommended for the diagnosis of diabetes, only for management and control.

The table below compares HbA1c and average blood glucose levels.

Table 9.1: Comparison of HbA1c and Blood Glucose

Blood Glucose	HbA1c
90–100	5–6 (normal)
90–120	5–6 (good control)
150–180	6–8 (fair control)
180–270	8–11 (poor control)
270–360 or above	11–14 (very poor control)

Self-Monitoring of Blood Glucose Level with a Glucometer

At present glucometers that are small and convenient to use are available. They are battery operated and portable. With a simple finger prick with a lancet, blood is drawn onto a paper strip that has been inserted into the machine. Within minutes the blood sugar value is displayed on the screen. New models of glucometers that have dispensed with finger pricking and paper strips are also available.

GlucoWatch®

A new innovation called a GlucoWatch® (recently approved by the FDA) estimates glucose levels by using sensors. This eliminates the need to draw blood by finger pricks. This is extremely useful for children suffering from type 1 diabetes whose sugar levels need to be tested several times a day. It sounds an alarm when the child's glucose hits dangerously low or high levels, which can happen when the child is asleep.

Within minutes the blood glucose level is displayed on the screen. Such estimates help patients learn about their diabetic statuses more frequently and thus regulate their conditions. Such self-estimations are essential in the regulation and management of type 1 diabetes. For patients with type 1 diabetes, blood sugar levels have to be tested several times during the day because the patients are on insulin and need constant monitoring. For patients with type 2, it is advisable to test blood sugar levels twice a day after medication has been prescribed and standardized. The test should be done once fasting and then before lunch and/or dinner. If done only once, it is preferred to check the fasting glucose level. Some individuals check once a day, alternating fasting and prelunch timing.

Some authors recommend testing blood sugar levels more than twice a day. The paper strips used in the machines are expensive and should be used judiciously because the procedure will be performed throughout the patient's life. This is especially true for patients living in third world countries. Frequent testing adds to the cost of diabetic care, so the time and frequency of testing should be what is most beneficial to the patient.

If the results are not within the prescribed limits on repeated examination, a medical consultation becomes necessary. In a diabetic patient, the fasting blood glucose level should range between 90 mg percent and 120 mg percent. At one hour after a meal, the recommended value of blood glucose level is less than 180 mg percent; at two hours after a meal it should be between 140 mg percent and 160 mg percent.

While using glucose meters, the following precautions should be taken:
1. Use fresh glucose strips that are not discolored or expired.
2. Periodically calibrate the meter with control solution.

3. Keep the meter clean.
4. Periodically compare the meter results to laboratory results; the results should be within 15 percent of each other.
5. Replace the meter batteries regularly.

Close and regular contact with health-care professionals and ongoing self-education go a long way in helping the patient lead a healthy life.

Urine Test for Glucose

Patients can evaluate their diabetic statuses by testing urine instead of blood using the paper strip method. These strips are cheap and can be used more frequently without worrying about the cost. However, urine testing is becoming obsolete. The results of urine tests give only a rough estimate of the blood glucose levels, and sugar appears in urine only when the blood glucose level exceeds 180 mg percent. The urine sample gives no indication of the current status. This anomaly can be mitigated to some extent by using a double-voided urine sample. This method has become obsolete in the United States but is still prevalent in third world countries.

Double-voided urine sample means that at first, urine is completely voided, and after about fifteen minutes another urine sample is collected and tested.

The advantage of urine testing is that it is cheap, and if the test is positive on repeated examinations it surely indicates uncontrolled diabetes mellitus.

Urine ketone testing still remains an important procedure in patients with type 1 diabetes and those with gestational diabetes. Self-monitoring of blood glucose levels is as important as planning meals, daily physical activity at one's place of work, medication, and exercise. Keeping accurate records of the results of blood glucose levels and daily routines helps patients regulate their diabetes scientifically rather than depending on guesswork.

Hyperglycemia Due to Other Causes

Besides diabetes there are many causes of hyperglycemia. These include tumors and nontumorous conditions of the adrenal and pituitary glands and certain disorders of the liver. These conditions should be considered in the differential diagnosis of diabetes. A number of other hormones produced in the body have actions opposite to that of insulin, and different glands produce these hormones.

Table 9.2: Causes of Hyperglycemia

Name of tumor or condition	Hormone produced
Glucagon-secreting tumor of the pancreas	Glucagons, with action opposite to insulin
Cushing's syndrome of the adrenal gland	Cortisone; causes hyperglycemia
Prolactin-secreting tumor of the pituitary gland	Prolactin; blocks insulin action
Acromegaly	Growth hormone; blocks insulin sensitivity
Pheochromocytoma of the adrenal gland	Adrenaline; causes hyperglycemia
Hyperthyroidism	Thyroxine; causes glucose intolerance
Stomatostatin-secreting tumor of the pancreas	Stomatostatin; blocks insulin secretion by islet cells

CHAPTER 10

Pregnancy and Alcohol

Some things don't mix

This chapter describes the precautions to take and rules to follow when diabetes is associated with pregnancy. The perverse fascination with alcoholic drinks and a decline in simple living has driven people away from nature and made them prey to ailments, especially those with diabetes.

The most fulfilling experience of modern innovations is saving the babies of pregnant women with diabetes. One heart-rending incident comes to mind. It occurred nearly fifty years ago, when I was posted in a maternity ward as an intern. A full-term diabetic woman had been admitted, and she had conceived after several years of marriage. It was a premature delivery, and unfortunately the baby died at birth. The mother and father were devastated.

Several years ago diabetic women could not conceive; repeated stillbirths and miscarriages were the order of the day. Today pregnancies can be planned and carried to full term, and parents can rejoice.

Diabetes in Pregnant Women

For women with diabetes, a pregnancy has to be planned well before conception. Some nondiabetic women develop diabetes during pregnancy—this is known as gestational diabetes mellitus (GDM). They require as much meticulous care during pregnancy as their diabetic companions.[65]

Rigid criteria have been established for screening GDM, and glucose tolerance tests are done to determine risk levels. Depending on specific population groups, abnormal glucose tolerance occurs in 3 to 10 percent of pregnancies. Incidence of GDM is 1.5 to 2 percent in white Americans and 5 to 8 percent in Hispanics, African-Americans, and Asians. The frequency is higher in Native Americans (up to 15 percent).

To detect GDM, screening tests are done in the first trimester. The tests are more pertinent in the following instances:
- The mother is older than thirty-five.
- She previously had a large baby.
- There is an unexplained death of a previous baby.
- There is a family history of diabetes.
- The mother is obese.
- She had high blood glucose levels in a previous pregnancy

Precautions before Conception

Before a woman conceives, she must control her diabetes. It is recommended that her HbA1C should be less than 7 percent, preferably closer to 6 percent. If she is obese, she must lose weight, and she should be examined for kidney or eye complications because these are aggravated during pregnancy. Blood sugar must be rigidly controlled to create a healthy environment for conception.

When a diabetic woman becomes pregnant, she has to take extra precautions to manage her diabetes. During the pregnancy high blood sugar can harm both her and the baby.

Diabetic Nephropathy Advances If Glycemic Control Is Poor

During pregnancy oral antidiabetic drugs are contraindicated; they harm the baby and are to be strictly avoided. The drug of choice is insulin, and a pregnant mother should be fully versed in its use. The amount of insulin given is carefully monitored because the nutritional demand on the mother increases as her pregnancy advances, and the dose has to be adjusted along with her diet to maintain a steady balance. With the growth of the placenta, a surge of placental hormones induces insulin resistance. Six meals should be eaten per day. Blood glucose levels should be checked several times during the day, and hypoglycemia and hyperglycemia should be avoided at all costs. Her glucose profile should be a meticulous replication of a healthy woman's to avoid morbidities (deadly complications), such as abortion. There is an increased tendency for hypoglycemia, which should be avoided by keeping a snack at hand. Exercise is a must, but it should never be rigorous.

During pregnancy high blood sugar levels can harm the mother as well as the baby, and eye and other complications can develop or get worse if they are already present. Diabetic nephropathy[66] advances if blood glucose control is poor. Maternal morbidity is high, and hypertension and preeclampsia take their tolls. Besides miscarriage and birth defects, large babies form. Strict blood sugar control before conception and during pregnancy decreases the incidence of birth defects by 1 to 5 percent while uncontrolled diabetes mellitus increases birth anomalies by four to eight times.

Diabetic nephropathy is a disease of kidneys that ultimately leads to end-stage failure of the kidneys.

A pregnant woman must keep certain things in mind:
- She must monitor her blood sugar daily (if necessary more than twice a day).
- A daily urine examination for ketone bodies is mandatory because pregnant women with diabetes are predisposed to ketoacidosis.
- Oral glucose-lowering agents are not recommended.
- The dose of insulin will need to be adjusted as pregnancy advances; as food intake increases, the dose of insulin must increase.
- Her meal plans and calorie requirements should be worked out carefully.
- She must have regular consultations with her health-care provider.
- She must abstain from alcohol, drugs, and smoking.
- The use of artificial sweeteners is not recommended.
- A good snack must always be kept handy in case of hypoglycemia, which tends to occur more often in pregnancy.
- Hyperglycemia leads to fat babies, which lead to fat kids, which lead to fat teenagers, which lead to fat adults.

Large Babies

Large babies (those who weigh 4,000 grams or more) develop when high blood sugar in the mother's blood passes into the baby's circulation and stimulates the pancreas to produce more insulin. The overactive pancreatic state extends into the early neonatal period, causing complications. The increased secretion of insulin in the neonatal period changes excess sugar into fat, which gets stored in the baby, making it overweight.

Fetal obesity develops a unique pattern of growth with deposits of excessive fat in the central abdomen and interscapular region (the area between the shoulder blades). Fetal birth weight correlates more with postprandial (after-meal) blood sugar than fasting levels. Accelerated growth thus stimulated often extends into childhood and adulthood. Fetal overgrowth causes hypoxia (a low oxygen level in the blood), resulting in defects in the cardiovascular and central nervous systems.

A large baby makes delivery difficult and may necessitate cesarean section. It may also induce premature labor and is susceptible to hypoglycemia soon after birth due to the overactive pancreas. The biophysical profile of the baby needs regular monitoring during pregnancy, and the time and route of delivery should be carefully evaluated during the last trimester. When the mother's blood sugar levels are within normal range, a baby of normal size develops.

Diabetes and Alcohol

There are contradictory views regarding how much alcohol people with diabetes should drink. Some permit a moderate intake (no more than two drinks per day for men and one per day for women) when diabetes is under complete control. One drink is equivalent to twelve ounces of beer, five ounces of wine, or one and a half ounces of distilled spirits. Others recommend total restrictions of smoking and drinking.

Drinking and smoking do not confer any health benefits but have definite harmful effects. Chronic alcohol abuse damages the pancreas, depleting its capacity to form and secrete insulin. Alcohol affects diabetic control and causes chaos with blood sugar levels. It can produce hyperglycemia as well as life-threatening hypoglycemia. It disturbs the lipid profile, raises triglyceride levels, and increases blood pressure, thereby increasing the risk of cardiac complications.

A patient should totally refrain from drinking alcohol if he or she has or is:
1. Pancreatitis.
2. Kidney dysfunction.
3. Lipid disorders.
4. Pregnant.
5. Overweight.
6. Given to alcoholic abuse.
7. Taking high doses of insulin and at risk of developing hypoglycemia.
8. Fever or any infectious disease.
9. In the recovery phase of any physical injury or trauma.

CHAPTER 11

The Pathogenesis of Diabetes

*It's far more important to know what person the disease
has than what disease the person has.*
- Hippocrates

This chapter describes the role of the cardiovascular system
in preserving the interior milieu and the changes that take
place when a person develops diabetes.[67] It discusses the consequences of these changes and their roles in the development of
complications. It also describes how the deposition of bad cholesterol (LDL) into the blood vessel walls compromises blood
circulation and how antioxidants affect the genesis of atherosclerosis. Antioxidants are substances that prevent oxygenation
of substances to form harmful chemicals, such as superoxides.

The body is made of tissues that are made of billions of cells, the
basic units of organic life. The cells are arranged in columns,
layers, and bundles to form organs. These cells are constantly
bathed in tissue fluid that separates them from one another and
flows like a stream around them. This fluid separates them from
blood vessels and is the medium through which each cell gets
food in the form of glucose as well as water and oxygen (which
is needed to burn glucose to release energy and sustain life). As

the cells perform their functions, waste is generated and must be removed from the system. The cells throw their waste into the tissue fluid.

The body has a system to reach the tissue fluid and fulfill the cells' requirements. The circulatory system fulfills the basic needs of the body with the help of other systems, including the liver, lungs, and kidneys. The circulatory, or cardiovascular, system is made of the heart and blood vessels, which are a lengthy system of pipelines that measures on average sixty thousand miles. These pipes spread like roads and lanes, and they reach every cell of the body. The blood vessels are further classified into arteries and veins. The arteries carry blood away from the heart, and the veins bring the blood back to the heart. The arteries are of three types: large, elastic arteries; medium-size muscular arteries; and small arteries and smaller vessels called capillaries. The large arteries are like highways; the medium-size arteries are like roads that run into organs; and the capillaries are like lanes that enter every house or cell in the body.

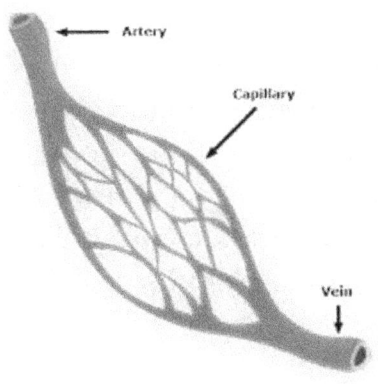

Capillary meshwork[68]

The veins drain away the arterial blood that flows into the capillaries, which are thin and form a network between the arteries and veins. They pass through the tissue fluid, and substances are exchanged between the tissue fluid and capillaries. For example, oxygen within the capillaries passes into the tissue fluid. It is picked up by the cells, and carbon dioxide (which is waste) flows from the cells into the tissue fluid and is carried away by the capillaries. In a similar manner other substances, like glucose, are exchanged between cells and capillaries.

The Heart

The heart pumps blood into the large blood vessels; it is then carried to the capillaries. The heart pumps hundreds of thousands of times every day, which is an enormous task. As blood pools into the capillary meshwork, the nutrients and oxygen ooze out of the capillaries, pass into the tissue fluid, and go into the cells. The waste is picked up by the capillaries from the tissue fluid, and the fluid is then taken back to the heart via the veins.

From the heart the blood goes to the lungs, which remove carbon dioxide and replenish the blood with oxygen. The blood flows through every organ of the body, delivering nutrients and removing waste. When blood flows through the kidneys, the kidneys remove other toxic wastes. The liver removes most chemicals, which are ultimately discarded as urine with the help of the kidneys.

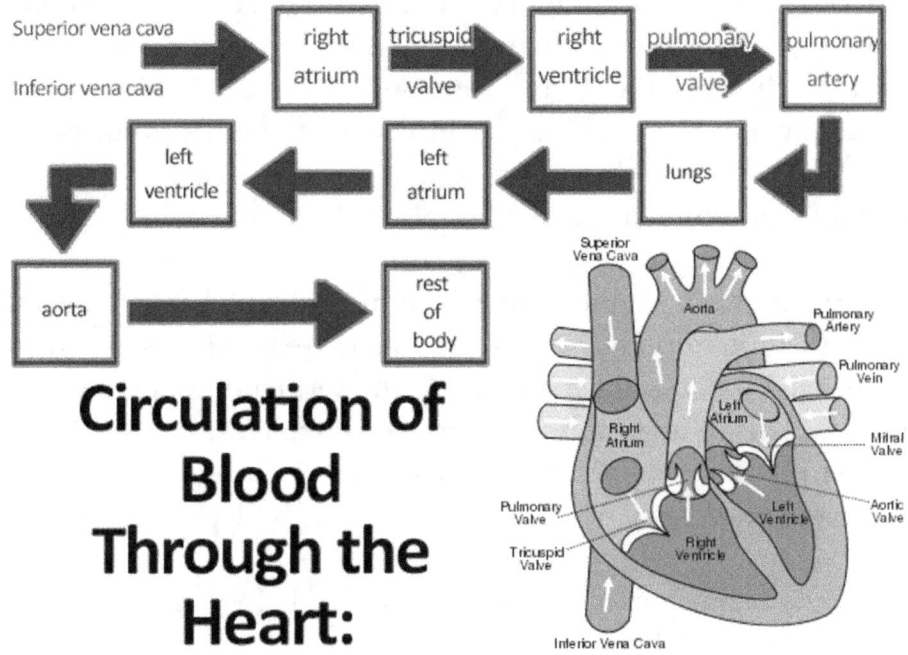

Circulation of blood through the heart [69]

A healthy body requires healthy cells, and for the cells to remain healthy it is vital that the cardiovascular system, the primary delivery network, remains disease free and efficient. The heart's pumping action, which pushes blood into the blood vessels, is achieved through the alternate contraction and relaxation of the muscle cells. The further flow of blood through the blood vessel network is achieved partly by the recoil of elastic vessels and partly by the contractile activity of muscular vessels.

Hypercholesterolemia

Any clog in the pipeline, or blood vessels, will obstruct the free flow of blood and seriously impair the delivery system. These clogs generally form when blood clots inside the lumen (hollow core) of a vessel. A tendency toward increased blood clotting is subsequent to the formation of cholesterol plaques on the inside of the vessel walls and the consequent thickening of the walls. Any damage to the inner linings of the walls predisposes the formation of cholesterol plaques and increases the tendency of clot formations within the lumen of the blood vessels.

These cholesterol plaques inside the lumen of blood vessels narrow the vessels and impair blood circulation. Increased levels of cholesterol in the blood predispose one to the formation of cholesterol plaques. This in turn causes arteriosclerosis and an increased tendency for blood clots within the walls. (*Arteriosclerosis* means thickening and hardening of the vessels, resulting in hypertension).

Hypercholesterolemia, arteriosclerosis, and clogging of the vessels are closely linked.

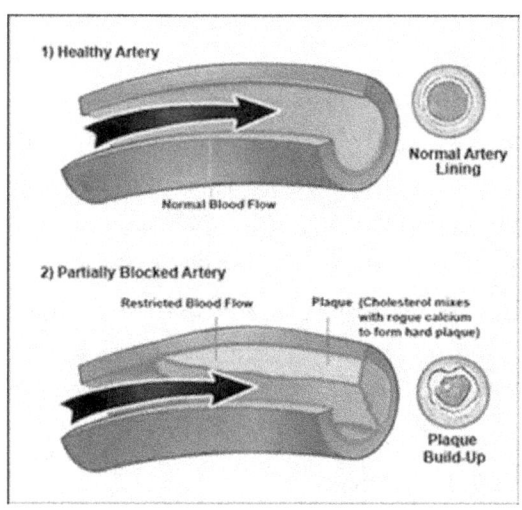

Hypercholesterolemia, cholesterol plaques, hypertension, clot formation, and vessel block [70]

Any damage to the muscle cells of the heart will adversely affect cardiovascular activity. Persons with diabetes are more prone to arteriosclerosis because their cholesterol levels are high, and their circulation is often compromised. The vessels supplying blood to the muscles of the heart, called coronary vessels, may also be affected, and in such a situation the cells of the heart are damaged.

Natural wear and tear goes on in the body, and the body can repair itself, but its ability is limited. Cells like neurons in the brain and spinal cord, once damaged, do not regenerate. Pancreatic islet cells, if damaged, are lost forever, as are the muscle cells of the heart.

In contrast the cells of the skin and the cells lining the cavities of hollow organs and tubelike structures such as the blood vessels have tremendous power to multiply and replenish lost cell mass. If the lining cells of a blood vessel are damaged at a higher rate, which frequently happens in persons with diabetes, the process of arteriosclerosis is hastened. Vitamins, especially vitamin C, are important for healing.

In a person with diabetes, blood glucose levels are high; the cells are starved because glucose is unable to enter due to the lack of or insensitivity to insulin. As a result their ability to repair suffers.

Two factors hasten the process of arteriosclerosis in diabetics: a high level of cholesterol in the blood and a higher rate of damage to the linings of the vessel walls.

For people with diabetes, besides impaired circulation due to arteriosclerosis, which impairs the nutrition of the cells, glucose is not available to the cells due to a lack of insulin.

In a diabetic patient, high glucose in the blood forms an insoluble complex (AGE; see below) with proteins present in the blood. This complex tends to get deposited on the insides of the vessel walls and occludes them. This seriously impairs circulation, especially microcirculation (circulation of blood in capillaries), which further compromises the nutrition of the cells.

Advanced glycosylation end (AGE) products are formed when blood glucose binds with different proteins in the blood, creating insoluble compounds that tend to deposit on the blood vessel walls, thereby narrowing the lumina of the vessels.

In response to a lack of use of glucose, the fats are mobilized from adipose (fat) tissue, thrown into the blood, and taken to the liver, which metabolizes the fats and throws them back into the circulating blood. The resulting high levels of LDL in the blood are harmful because they are closely linked to atherosclerosis and arteriosclerosis.

Atherosclerosis

Atherosclerosis (*athero* means "plaque"; *sclerosis* means "hardening") is a disease of the large and medium-size blood vessels. It is an ageing process that affects both the elderly and the young, though its seeds are implanted early in life. In this condition plaques made of cholesterol develop on the walls of blood vessels, narrowing and constricting them. The cholesterol comes from the blood stream. LDL cholesterol forms the plaques, but before its entry into the vessel walls it is oxidized (oxygen is added) and picked up by macrophages (the scavenger cells of the body), which exist in the walls of blood vessels. In this way LDL is deposited in the plaques.

It is not known why LDL is so closely associated with athero-sclerosis. When the level of LDL in the blood is high, the level of HDL is low in an almost inverse ratio. HDL is a protective fat that helps lower the risk of arteriosclerosis (see below). The level of LDL cholesterol is high in diabetics, making them more prone to atherosclerosis. The prerequisite for the deposition of LDL in the vessel walls is its oxidation. Antioxidants in meals help hinder oxidation and reduce the formation of atheroscle-rotic plaques.

Arteriosclerosis

Arteriosclerosis is a disease that affects many blood vessels but chiefly the coronary and carotid vessels. The coronary vessels nourish the heart muscle. When circulation in the coronary arteries is compromised due to temporary spasms of the vessels, the oxygen supply to the muscle cells of the heart decreases, and the patient feels pain or constriction in the chest, which is called angina. When a coronary vessel is occluded by a blood clot, a portion of the heart that is deprived of oxygen undergoes degeneration, resulting in a heart attack. A similar situation can occur in carotid arteries (blood vessels carrying blood to the brain) and lead to stroke.

In obese persons the fat cells inside the abdominal cavity pro-duce a substance called plasminogen activator inhibitor-1. This substance prevents the dissolution of clots within the blood vessels and thereby predisposes a person to heart attacks and strokes. Therefore obese persons are at greater risk of coronary disease and stroke.

When the blood supply to the kidneys is compromised, degen-erative changes take place in the kidneys. They start to produce a substance called angiotensin, which raises blood pressure. High blood pressure, or hypertension, is a common complication of diabetes, and it further aggravates arteriosclerosis.

The lining cells of the blood vessels (endothelial cells) are dysfunctional in persons with diabetes. As a result the proper dilatation of the blood vessels suffers.

Physiological Malfunctioning in Diabetes

In a diabetic patient, the circulation of blood in the vessels is compromised due to three factors:

- Increased incidence of arteriosclerosis.
- Deposition of protein-glucose complex inside the vessel walls.
- Endothelial cell dysfunction, resulting in decreased vasodilatation (expansion of the blood vessels).

The impaired circulation affects the nutrition of the cells and compromises the functioning of every organ and system. As the nutrition of the nervous system suffers, neurological symptoms such as numbness, tingling, burning, and loss of sensations in the hands and feet and sciatica-type pain occur. Sciatica is shooting pain in the back of the leg.

Higher Rate of Infection

When the immune system is at low ebb, serious infections can occur, and the patient takes longer to overcome them.

The patient often can miss a small cut on a foot due to the loss of sensation. Because of poor vitality of the skin and underlying tissues, the wound refuses to heal, leading to a nonhealing wound, and the infection may advance to a point where it necessitates amputation.

Excessive Hunger, Thirst, and Urination

A diabetic patient presents symptoms of excessive thirst, hunger, and urination. The person's blood sugar level is high, often above 180 mg percent. Whenever the level exceeds 180 mg percent, sugar spills into the urine in the kidney tubules. This raises the osmotic pressure of the urine, and the kidney tubules suck water from the blood to balance the pressure. More urine is formed, resulting in increased urination. This leads to dehydration, and the patient feels thirsty.

Osmotic pressure is the pressure of molecules (glucose) in fluid exerted across a semipermeable membrane.

Due to the inability to use glucose, the patient also feels hungry.

Ketosis

The brain depends largely on glucose for its energy needs, and when glucose is not available because it is low or because insulin is low, the person feels dizzy and may even faint. Due to the lack of glucose utilization, fats are mobilized into the circulation in the form of ketone bodies. The excess accumulation of ketone bodies causes ketosis, which is a life-threatening condition.

Weight Loss

Due to a lack of the use of glucose, body fat is broken down to meet energy demands, resulting in weight loss. The body also breaks down muscle proteins, and the person becomes lean.

The Somogyi Effect

Somogyi was a Hungarian scientist who described this effect—a rebound phenomenon in which the body reacts to extremely low blood sugar levels by overcompensating, resulting in high levels. When blood glucose falls, which sometimes happens in the middle of the night, the body secretes counter-regulatory hormones such as glucagon and epinephrine. Glucagon is a hormone secreted by the alpha cells present in the islets of Langerhans in the pancreas. The action of this hormone is opposite that of insulin. Epinephrine (or adrenaline) is secreted by the adrenal glands, which are found close to the kidneys. This hormone also raises blood sugar levels.

These hormones make the liver convert glycogen (present in its stores) into glucose and pour it into the blood, thereby raising blood glucose levels. This happens when the night dose of insulin is greater than required or the person's intake of food at dinner is less. The Somogyi effect can be avoided by proper doses of insulin and proper meal planning.

CHAPTER 12

Complications of Diabetes

Not something to be taken lightly

The death rate and gravity of complications of diabetes are so profound that no message is strong enough. The more you know about them the better.

An outline of lipid disorders, hypertension, heart attack, stroke, blindness, kidney failure, and numerous neuropathies is given in this chapter. Dental complications, nonhealing wounds, impaired immunity, and skin disorders are also discussed as well as problems that require immediate hospitalization.[71,72]

Serious complications include heart attack, hypertension, blindness, life-threatening infections, kidney failure, nonhealing wounds, and amputation. The benefits of rigid control of diabetes last for years, according to a recent follow-up study by the DCCT of the National Institute of Health (NIH).[73] The tight control of diabetes and continuing medical assessment of the patient delays the onset of eye and kidney complications. Researchers who conducted the United Kingdom Prospective Diabetic Study (UKPDS) have given substantial evidence that strict glycemic control can delay or prevent the onset of complications.[74]

The prevention of complications remains an important element in the total management of diabetes. Recognizing the factors that induce complications and correctly carrying out instructions will go a long way in decreasing complications. Self-care, awareness, and vigilance in such situations will help reduce morbidity and death rate.

Lipid Disorders

All diabetic patients, young and old, must have their lipid profiles evaluated at the time of diagnosis and at regular intervals. In adults LDL cholesterol should be less than 100 mg percent; HDL cholesterol should be greater than 45 mg percent, and triglycerides should be less than 200 mg percent.

Thyroid disorders, such as hypothyroidism, can elevate lipid levels. These may coexist with diabetes and should be ruled out. Thyroid hormone deficiency should be corrected.

The Scandinavian Simvastatin Survival Study demonstrated[75,76,77] that the use of simvastatin, a cholesterol-lowering drug, resulted in a 35 percent decrease on average of LDL cholesterol and reduced coronary mortality (death due to heart attack) by 42 percent. Coexisting conditions and disorders, such as smoking, hypertension, premature coronary heart disease (CHD), and familial hypercholesterolemia, should be taken into consideration while targeting lipid levels. Statins are generally well tolerated, and so they are the first line of action in treating diabetic dyslipidemia (abnormal blood lipid levels).[78] When triglyceride levels are high, fibric acid derivatives (compounds with medicinal use) may be used. These are another class of lipid-lowering drugs. When using a combination of therapies, such as fibric acid plus statins, it is recommended that low doses of statins be used because they have been found to be safer.

Coronary Heart Disease and Hypertension

Patients with diabetes are at higher risk of developing high blood pressure (hypertension). It is estimated that 60 to 65 percent of patients with diabetes develop hypertension, which further raises the risk of heart disease,[79] which is already high in diabetics; it also increases the risk of diabetic retinopathy.

UKPDS trials showed that hypertension was associated with an increased risk of all complications, and the tight control of blood pressure decreased the overall risk by nearly 24 percent in all end-stage conditions linked with diabetes. Hypertension accelerates arteriosclerosis and decreases blood supply to the tissues, so it is important to control blood pressure rigidly. The UKPDS group also revealed that blood pressure control decreased the risk of stroke in patients with type 2 diabetes. It demonstrated that improved blood pressure control resulted in a 44 percent reduction in the risk of fatal and nonfatal strokes.

The ADA recommends all patients with diabetes ensure their blood pressure is less than 130 mm/Hg (mercury) systolic and 85 mm/Hg diastolic. Investigations and surveys at the National Center for Chronic Disease Prevention and Health Promotion and the Centers for Disease Control and Prevention have shown that the control of hypertension in United States is not adequate. The investigators concluded that 71 percent of adult diabetics had high blood pressure. The incidence increased with age and was elevated in both sexes as well as in non-Hispanic blacks and non-Hispanic whites. Of all the persons with elevated blood pressure, only 71 percent were aware of their condition, and only 57 percent were treating it. Control of blood pressure was least common among elderly patients.[80]

The heartbeat is the rhythmic contraction and relaxation of the heart muscle. When it contracts it pushes blood into blood vessels, and the pressure measured at that time is named systolic blood pressure. When the heart relaxes, the blood pressure measured in the blood vessels is called diastolic.

Just as it is important to control blood sugar, it is equally important to control blood pressure. Patients whose blood pressure is controlled have reduced risks of heart attack, stroke, and angina. Regular checkups of blood pressure are essential. Smoking and alcohol tend to raise blood pressure, especially in people who are already predisposed, such as diabetics. Mild hypertension can be controlled by simple measures, such as controlling body weight, reducing alcohol and smoking, and decreasing intake of salt. If these measures fail or if the hypertension is marked, medical consultation and medication may be required.

Antihypertensive Drugs

Angiotensin converting enzyme (ACE) inhibitors are antihypertensive agents. They have been found to be effective and well tolerated. They have favorable effects in reducing microalbuminuria (the loss of albumin in urine exceeding 30 mg per day) and nephropathy. They have no adverse effects on glucose or insulin levels, and some studies show improved insulin sensitivity. ACE inhibitors are contraindicated for pregnant women.[81]

Other antihypertensive drugs such as beta-blockers and calcium channel blockers are effective. Salt restriction and a low-fat diet are strongly recommended. Compared to nondiabetic subjects, heart disease appears earlier in life in diabetics. It affects men and women alike and is more often fatal. Deaths due to heart attack are 20 percent more likely in diabetics compared to nondiabetic patients. Seventy to eighty percent of diabetic adults die of coronary artery disease, stroke, or peripheral vascular disease. This incidence is two to four times greater than for nondiabetic adults.

Rigid control of blood glucose levels and blood pressure significantly reduces the risk of these complications. The incidence of repeat heart attack is greater in diabetics compared to nondiabetics, and the most common cause of death in adults with diabetes is coronary disease. About 9 percent of diabetic adults suffer from stroke.

The thickening and narrowing that takes place in the coronary blood vessels also takes place in the blood vessels of the brain. Heart attack and stroke occur due to the decrease of blood supplies to these vital organs. The decrease is due to thickening and rigidity of the walls of the blood vessels as well as the narrowing of their lumina, which results when fats are deposited on the walls of the vessels. If blood clots within these narrowed vessels, the result is complete blockage.

High levels of LDL cholesterol and triglycerides contribute to this process. Several studies have revealed that lipid-lowering drugs reduce the incidence of coronary artery disease. The data also showed that treating diabetic patients with simvastatin lowered the incidence of coronary events in hyperlipidemic cases by 55 percent.

The Cholesterol and Recurrent Events (CARE) study revealed that pravastatin,[82] another cholesterol-lowering drug, was effective in reducing the risk of coronary artery disease (CAD) by 25 percent in patients with diabetes and 23 percent in patients without diabetes. One aspirin tablet of 75 to 150 mg, taken daily, helps to prevent clotting and goes a long way in the prevention of heart attacks. This is to be taken with medical consultation.

Lower Extremity Arterial Disease (LEAD)

LEAD is identified by an absence of or a deficit in the peripheral pulses in the lower legs and feet. This represents decreased blood supply and reduced arterial perfusion (circulation) of the extremities, and it causes intermittent claudication (pain in the leg while walking that disappears on resting). In population-based studies, pulse deficits were found in 10 percent of diabetic adults, and 20 to 30 percent of cases were absent pulses. About 9 percent of diabetics suffered from intermittent claudication. The incidence increases with age, longer duration of diabetes, cigarette smoking, hypertension, and dyslipidemia.[83]

LEAD aggravates the situation when compounded with peripheral neuropathy and an increased susceptibility to infection.

Insulin Resistance Syndrome

Insulin resistance syndrome (IRS) is also known as syndrome X or CHOAS (which stands for coronary artery disease, hypertension, obesity, atherosclerosis, and stroke). The exact genesis of insulin resistance has not been elucidated. One theory is that high levels of fatty acids in the blood circulation of obese individuals block insulin receptors on tissue cells and cause insulin resistance.[84,85] IRS could have a genetic basis.

It is a vicious cycle: high levels of insulin cause obesity because insulin favors lipogenesis, and obesity produces insulin resistance and increased insulin production by the pancreas.

Another theory proposes that a PC1 protein interferes with the normal functioning of insulin receptors. The level of this protein is higher in people with type 2 diabetes compared to healthy persons. Its synthesis is genetically determined.

This syndrome is associated with obese persons with type 2 diabetes, and it sometimes presents in persons even before the disease is recognized and the diagnosis is established. Such individuals, besides being obese, are characterized by high levels of insulin in the blood. This is also seen in persons with IGT. This syndrome is also associated with hyperlipidemia, hyperinsulinemia, hypertension, coronary disease, and stroke.

IRS is seen in many adults in the United States. Smoking, lack of exercise, and high consumption of carbohydrates predispose people to IRS. Controlling body weight, changing a sedentary lifestyle, eating fewer fats and cholesterol, and adequate control of diabetes help in decreasing insulin resistance and alleviating the risk of complications.[86]

Diabetic Eye Disease

Eye and vision disturbances such as the following are common in diabetics:

- Loss of peripheral vision.
- Hazy vision.
- Floaters.
- Flashes or any visual disturbance.

These should be taken seriously. Visual disturbances call for immediate medical consultations.

A friend of mine came to me and complained that his vision had become hazy. When I tested his blood sugar, it was more than 300 mg percent. He had been careless in controlling his diet and diabetes, and the hazy vision frightened him. An ophthalmologist reported that the visual defect was due to early cataract. He went on a diet and regularly monitored his blood sugar levels, and strict control of his diabetes hindered further progression of the disease.

Regular eye checkups are mandatory.

In uncontrolled diabetes, a number of eye problems can occur:
- Diabetic retinopathy.
- Cataract.
- Glaucoma.

Diabetic Retinopathy

Diabetic retinopathy[87,88] is the leading cause of blindness among American adults. Between twelve thousand and twenty-four thousand cases of blindness occur each year due to diabetic retinopathy. It is twice as common as cataract and glaucoma among persons with diabetes. The prevalence of this complication is strongly related to the duration of the illness. Nearly all people with type 1 diabetes develop retinopathy after twenty years, as do more than 60 percent of people with type 2 diabetes. Research has revealed that poor control of diabetes has a strong association with retinopathy. Strict control of blood glucose levels not only prevents but also delays the development and slows the progression of this complication.

In this condition the blood vessels of the retina (the innermost coat of the eyeball, with the photoreceptors that visualize light) undergo distortion, becoming narrow at some points and widened at others. As a result the permeability of the vessels is affected, causing abnormal exudation (flowing out) of plasma and hemorrhages into the retina. As a result of exudation into the macular area, macular edema (fluid accumulation) occurs. The macula in the retina is also called "the yellow spot," and this is the area of maximum visual acuity. Edema in the macular area adversely affects eyesight. The edema and hemorrhages in the retina may seriously impair visual acuity and lead to blindness. There is no pain, and the symptoms may not appear until the disease is fairly well advanced. The longer a person suffers from diabetes, the greater the chances of developing retinopathy.

Early detection of this condition can help reduce the incidence. It is imperative that patients have their eyes examined at least once a year. The pupils should be dilated to permit the complete viewing of the inner chamber of the eye.

Laser treatment has decreased the incidence of severe visual impairment by nearly 60 percent.

Cataract

Cataract means clouding or opacification of the lens of the eye. High blood glucose levels lead to glucose oozing into the lens substance, where it forms a complex with the lens proteins. This is an insoluble compound, and it deposits into the lens substance. As a rule cataract develops as a part of the aging process. In diabetic patients it develops prematurely.

Glaucoma

Glaucoma indicates increased fluid pressure in the eyeball. The increased pressure on the retina and optic nerve leads to optic nerve atrophy (destruction or loss of tissue) and impairment of vision. The fluid is formed from the capillary channels in the eye. This fluid maintains the shape of the eyeball, and its excessive accumulation in the chamber of the eyeball causes glaucoma.

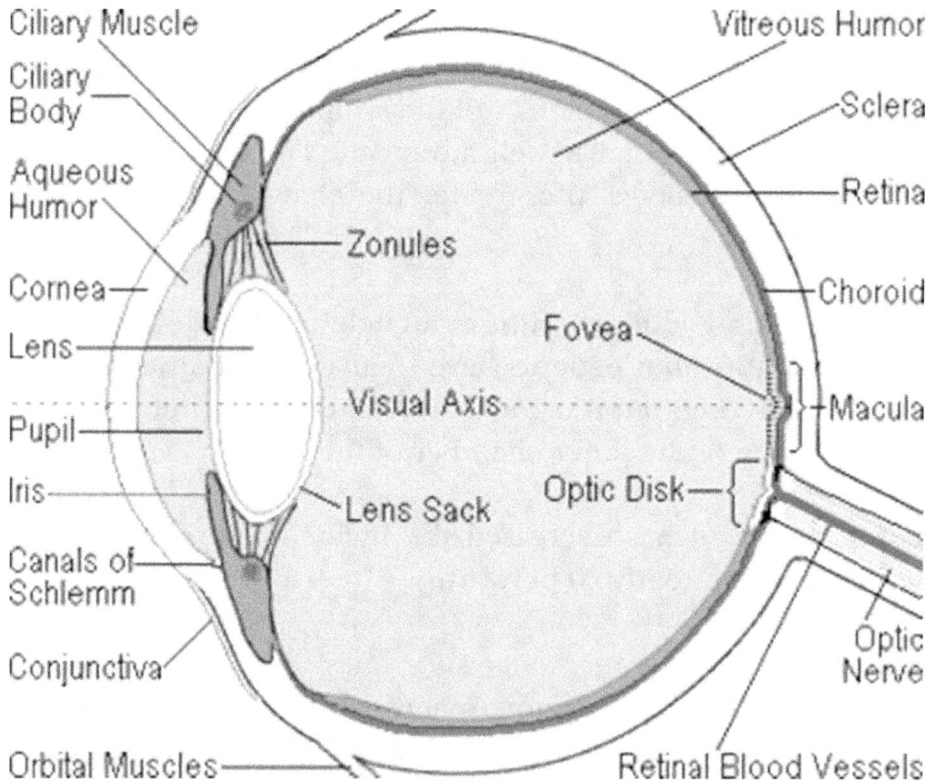

Horizontal section of the eyeball[89]

Kidney Disease

The ADA has reported that in the United States, more than twenty thousand patients with diabetes are diagnosed with end-stage renal disease (ESRD) every year.[90] Diabetes is the most common cause of ESRD. It is more common in African-Americans and Native Americans for reasons unknown. As shown by DCCT and UKPDS trials, intensive control of blood glucose in patients significantly reduces the risk of kidney damage and prevents or delays ESRD.

Symptoms of kidney disease or nephropathy usually occur in the late stages of the disease, when kidney function has fallen to 25 percent of normal. The earliest clinical sign of nephropathy is microalbuminuria. The loss of greater than 300 mg of albumin per day is present in frank nephropathy. ESRD develops in 50 percent of people with type 1 diabetes in ten years and in 75 percent by twenty years. Twenty to forty percent of people with type 2 diabetes progress to overt nephropathy if specific intervention is not provided. In 20 percent of type 2 diabetes cases, ESRD develops within twenty years.

Kidney Function Tests

The blood supplies to the kidneys are compromised over time due to the narrowing of blood vessels. This change occurs more often in type 1 diabetes than in type 2, and the changes are more marked and appear earlier.

Kidney function tests should be carried out from time to time after nephropathy has been detected. When nephropathy develops the patient should adhere to the following guidelines:
- A low-protein diet is advocated.
- Strict glycemic control is mandatory.

- If hypertension coexists, it should be treated seriously and adequately.
- Lipid levels should be rigidly controlled.

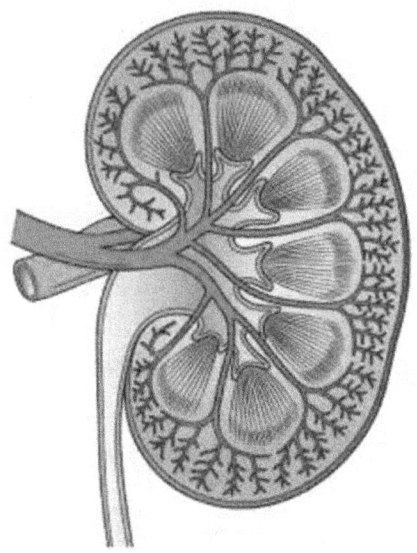

Cross section of human kidney[91]

The Structure of the Kidney

The functional unit of the kidney, called the nephron, is made up of the glomerulus and the tubules. The glomerulus consists of a meshwork of tiny blood vessels that filter the blood brought to the kidney by larger vessels. It removes body waste, which flows down the renal tubules. By virtue of its filtration process and differential absorption in the tubules, not only is toxic waste is removed from the body, but the salt water balance and acid base equilibrium of the body are preserved. As the vessels of the glomerulus become thick and narrow over time, the filtration process is impaired. The earliest manifestation of glomerular damage is the presence of traces of albumin in the urine.

Albumin is a protein in the blood. With impairment of glomerular function, albumin begins to leak into the urine. Microalbuminuria is the earliest clinical sign of nephropathy (kidney disease). Loss of greater than 30 mg per day of albumin is considered microalbuminuria. As damage increases, more albumin is lost into the urine. The loss of protein in the urine may be massive or minute and leads to other metabolic abnormalities.

The degenerative changes in the kidney lead to the ultimate production of angiotensin by the tubules of the kidney. Angiotensin is the substance that causes hypertension. It also narrows the vessels of the glomerulus and aggravates the degenerative process. ACE inhibitor drugs are effective in decreasing the levels of angiotensin, lowering hypertension, and decreasing the damage to the glomerulus.

The recommended levels of blood pressure are 130/85 mm/ Hg or less. Degeneration of the kidney ultimately ends in kidney failure.

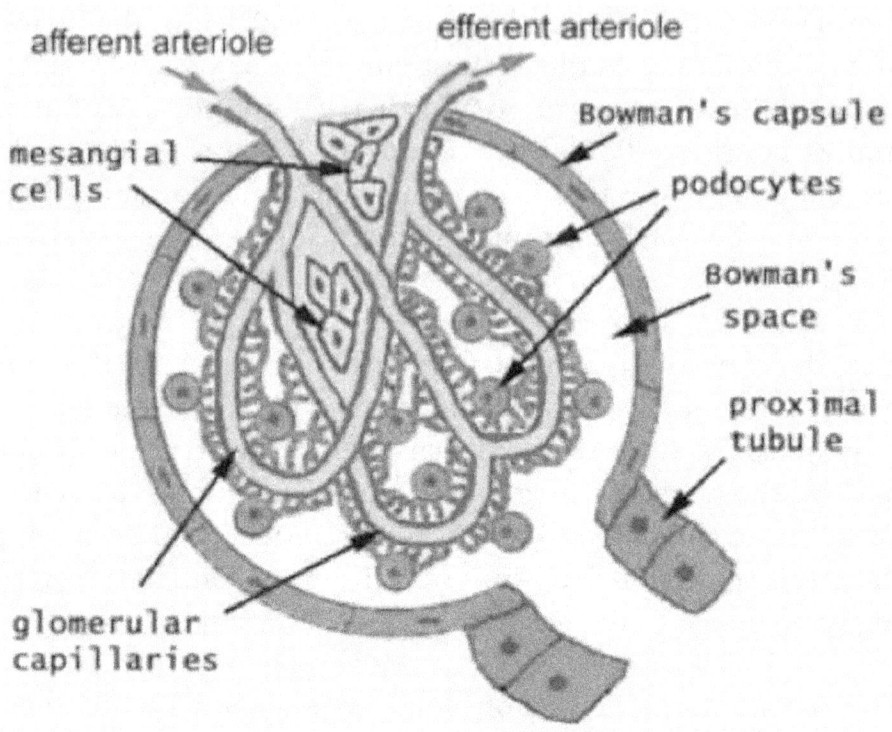

Structure of the glomerulus[92] [24]

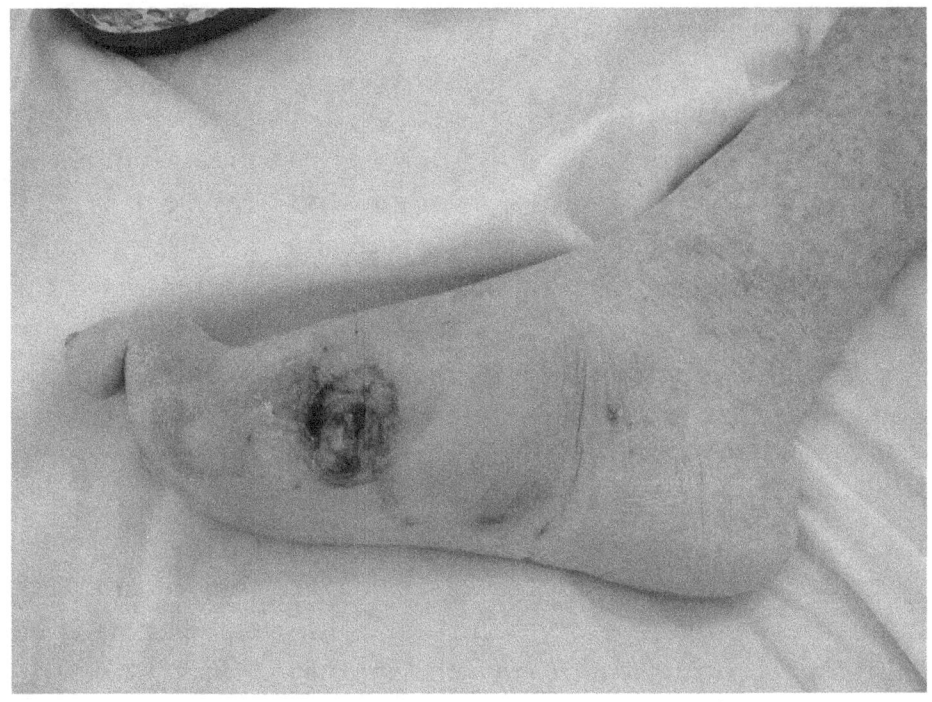

Foot ulcer[93]

A hammertoe is a toe that is bent because of a weakened muscle.

Foot ulcers are common in diabetics due to poor blood supply, low vitality of tissues, low immunity, and loss of sensations. They fail to heal and often lead to gangrene (decay and death of tissues in any part of the body).

Gangrene of the foot is twenty times more common among diabetics than matched controls, and this increased incidence is due to poor blood supply, neuropathy, and secondary infection. The decreased blood supply results from occlusion of micro and macro vessels. Cigarette smoking should be avoided because it aggravates the process. Once ulceration and gangrene set in, treatment is extremely difficult.

Diabetic Neuropathy

Diabetic neuropathy affects the nervous system, and about 60 percent of diabetic patients show some kind of nerve damage.[94] This is more common in patients with uncontrolled diabetes and in whom blood glucose levels have remained elevated for ten years or more. It can affect both types of diabetes patients. Alcohol and smoking increase the risk of developing diabetic neuropathy and can worsen an existing state of the condition. Strict glucose control may delay the progression or prevent the development of neuropathy.

Diabetic neuropathy can involve the sensory, motor, and autonomic nerves. The sensory and motor nerves belong to the voluntary nervous system, and the autonomic nerves belong to the involuntary nervous system. The voluntary nervous system supplies the skeletal muscles and the skin and is under the conscious control of the mind. The involuntary nervous system innervates the internal organs and is beyond the conscious control of the mind. Microangiopathy, a disease of small blood vessels in diabetes, results in decreased blood supplies to the nerves and damage to the nerves. The damage may also result from metabolic effects of diabetes. Some of these changes are reversible in the early stages if the diabetes is brought under control.

Sensory Disturbances

Sensory disturbances pertain to sensations in the body. There may be a loss of or decreased sensations or the feeling of abnormal sensations.

Distal Polyneuropathy

Distal means the involvement of the peripheral nerves, and *poly-neuropathy* means multiple nerve involvement. In this condition the distal portions of the limbs (the hands, feet, and adjoining portions of the arms and legs) are affected. The sensory system is the first to be affected, and the perceptions of pain, touch, and temperature become dull. Patients may feel abnormal sensations such as tingling, burning, or extreme cold in the hands or feet, or they may feel as if ants are crawling on them. They may feel as if they are walking on rocks or may not feel the firmness of the ground beneath their feet.

There may be a loss of balance and coordination, and the person's insensitivity to pain may be such that small cuts on the feet go unfelt and unnoticed. All these symptoms are worse at night.

Sometimes the involvement of the roots of the nerves results in excruciating pain in the area of distribution of the nerve supply.

Motor Disturbances

The damage to motor nerves, which innervate the muscles of the hands and feet, may cause weakness of the movements of the hands and feet. Involvement of some nerves can cause weakness of the muscles that move the eyeballs, resulting in diplopia (double vision). If the nerve supplying the muscles of the face is affected, the eyelids may droop, or the mouth may not close fully, and food may dribble out.

Focal neuropathy occurs most frequently in older patients. Specific nerves are affected, more often in the torso, head, and leg. The onset of symptoms is sudden and self-limiting. It can cause problems of hearing and even facial paralysis, difficulty in focusing, and double vision when the nerves of the head are involved. Severe pain in the lower back or pelvis, chest, stomach, and thigh may occur. Pain in the chest may mimic a heart attack.

Autonomic Disturbances

Autonomic neuropathy affects the nerves supplying the internal organs of the body. The damage to the autonomic nerves may cause the following symptoms:

1. Gastrointestinal disturbances, such as bouts of diarrhea and constipation. When the nerves of the stomach are involved, the stomach fails to empty in normal time. Food does not enter the intestine and hence is not digested on time. This results in brittle diabetes as the blood glucose levels fluctuate wildly; while antidiabetic drugs continue to be active, glucose fails to reach the bloodstream due to the delayed absorption.

2. Diarrhea may be severe (more than ten motions in a day).

3. The nerve damage to the muscles of the urinary bladder may result in an inability to empty the bladder completely. Due to loss of the sensation of bladder fullness and an inability to contract the bladder muscles, controlling the bladder and adequately and completely emptying it are lost. This results in stagnation of urine inside the bladder, which predisposes the patient to urinary tract infections.

4. Men may have difficulty attaining and maintaining erections. Women may not be able to achieve orgasm.

5. Postural hypotension (a sudden fall in blood pressure when standing up from a lying down position) can occur.

6. Lack of sweating may occur in the feet.

7. In the late stages, the heart may fail to speed up with exercise. Patients may not feel chest pain and thus have a heart attack without being aware of it.

8. Bile may stagnate in the gall bladder due to failure of the muscles of the bile passages to contract; this predisposes the formation of gallstones.

9. Patients may have difficulty sensing hypoglycemia.

Many drugs are available for the treatment of neurological complications. These include antidepressants, antiepileptics, and painkillers. Acupuncture has been tried as well as electrical stimulation of painful nerve endings.

Sexual Dysfunction

Sex and love intricately weave into our happiness. An unsatisfactory sex life leaves many distraught. Diabetics may face a number of sexual inadequacies and disturbances, but these can be handled. People with diabetes should not feel shy about or hesitate to discuss their problems with their doctors. They should not deny themselves basic instincts and pleasures.

Men often experience a lack of erections. This could be the result of vascular, neurological, or psychological reasons. Men feel fewer, less-firm erections that do not last long enough, and this may fail to arouse orgasms in his partner. Impotence often increases with age and the duration of diabetes. Excessive intake of alcohol, smoking, and drugs such as opiates also aggravate it. Intercourse can produce hypoglycemia, especially in men. It is good to have candy at hand.

Women often feel the absence of sexual desire. Beside diminished sexual response during intercourse, women may experience vaginal pain that may be aggravated by fungal infections. Increased vaginal dryness could be caused by a decrease in sex hormones with advancing age and the diabetic process.

All these conditions can be easily treated with medicines, but good blood sugar control underlines all therapies.

Impaired Immunity

Due to a depressed immune response, diabetic patients are more susceptible to infections. Studies conducted by NIH indicate the following:[95]

- Higher risk of surgical wound infection (as in hip replacements).
- Greater chance of reactivation of tuberculosis.
- Beta streptococcal infections.
- Higher mortality from influenza and pneumonia.
- Incidence of urinary tract infections in women with diabetes are higher compared to nondiabetic women.

Skin Diseases

A diabetic patient becomes predisposed to diseases of the skin, such as the following:

1. The patient is susceptible to both bacterial and fungal infections. A small cut or abrasion, if it gets infected, can develop into a boil or carbuncle and then it requires aggressive therapy. Fungal infections can develop between the toes, especially if the feet remain warm and moist.
2. Alopecia (loss of hair) can develop with type 1 diabetes.
3. Vitiligo (loss of healthy skin pigmentation) may develop with type 1 diabetes.
4. Diabetic patients can develop thick, dry skin.

5. Insulin hypertrophy (accumulation of fat at the site of insulin injections) can occur.

6. Insulin lipoatrophy (loss of fat at the site of insulin injections) can occur.

Dental Complications

Poor blood glucose control can result in gingivitis, tooth decay, and periodontal disease. The thickening of blood vessels in a diabetic patient reduces the blood supply to the gums, thereby reducing the supply of oxygen and vital nutrients. This decreases the resistance of the gums to infections. Moreover, the high levels of glucose in the environment allow the bacteria in the mouth to thrive.

When diabetes is poorly controlled, the high glucose levels in the mouth, added to the poor resistance of the gums, help bacteria proliferate and cause gingivitis; the gums become swollen, red, and painful. If untreated this will progress into periodontitis, which is infection and inflammation of the tissues around the teeth. The pocket of infection around the teeth may burrow deeper to infect the bony socket holding the teeth. The affected teeth may loosen and fall out.

To avoid dental complications and maintain good dental health, the patient should do the following:
- Avoid starchy foods that stick to the teeth.
- Regularly brush the teeth with a soft-bristled toothbrush in the morning and at bedtime.
- Clean between the teeth to remove plaques.
- Avoid chewing tobacco.

When the first sign of inflammation appears, such as gingivitis, consult a doctor.

Joint Problems

Osteoarthritis is common in old age. In a diabetic patient this degenerative disorder can be more common, can occur at an earlier age, and can be more severe. The joints become stiff and painful, with restricted mobility. This may result in deformities and formation of contractures as a result of thickened and contracted tendons and ligaments around the joints. The joints of the hands and feet may be affected, but the knee joints are the most commonly affected, and osteoarthritis of the knee joint is by far the most distressing. Surgery involving knee-joint replacement is often contemplated in such cases.

Painkillers are frequently taken for relief. Drugs that are toxic to the kidneys, such as nonsteroidal anti-inflammatory drugs, should be avoided. Regular and proper exercises designed for each joint are advocated.

Some acute complications of diabetes may require immediate attention and hospitalization.

Hypoglycemia

In hypoglycemia the blood sugar level falls below 60 mg percent, and the patient experiences extreme hunger, anxiety, palpitations, pallor, and cold, clammy sweating.[96,97] These symptoms are due to the secretion of adrenaline, which comes into action whenever blood glucose falls. The patient may also feel dizzy and experience a loss of concentration, confusion, fatigue, and headache (neuroglycopenic symptoms). If not corrected this leads to convulsions and coma.

Hypoglycemia occurs due to inadequate permeation of glucose into the brain cells. The condition is often precipitated by excessive intake of insulin, oral hypoglycemic drugs as sulfonyl-ureas, inadequate food intake, exercise, alcohol consumption, onset of menses, and the immediate postpartum period. It can occur in diabetic patients who rigidly control their conditions by overexercising and cutting down their food without adequately adjusting the doses of their antidiabetic drugs. Aspirin and other salicylates can lead to hypoglycemia by increasing the effects of antidiabetic drugs.

To correct this state, patients must eat candy or sugar cubes or drink orange juice. If they do not respond to these measures, they should be taken to a hospital. All diabetic patients should carry candy with them to deal with the dangerous situation of hypoglycemia.

Diabetic Ketoacidosis
This condition is an emergency that requires immediate medical attention and hospitalization. Diabetic ketoacidosis is an excess of ketone bodies in blood and urine. See page ninety-five.

Diabetic Coma
This condition is an emergency that requires immediate hospitalization.

PART 3

CHAPTER 13

Preventing Diabetes

What we think, we become.
—Gautama Buddha

This chapter discusses the necessary measures people can take to prevent diabetes. The seeds of diabetes are sown in the genes, but certain measures are within an individual's means and can delay or prevent the manifestation of diabetes.

An overview of the Diabetic Prevention Program (DPP) initiated and designed by the NIH is given in this chapter. A point-based system to determine the risk of diabetes and the research on Pima Indians and its outcome are mentioned. Drugs and lifestyle changes needed for the prevention of diabetes are discussed.

The secret to health lies in prevention. If a person is at high risk of developing diabetes, every effort should be made to delay or prevent its onset.

A simple measure is to get blood sugar tested on regular basis and detect IGT as early as possible. People should watch their weight. Checkups should be done yearly, especially of blood pressure, blood sugar, and serum cholesterol. This is with respect to type 2 diabetes, which is much more common than type 1.

The Onset of Diabetes

Patients must note when the disease is in the dormant phase (it can be called the prediabetic stage). At this stage the person may show IGT. The disease may spin out of control and precipitate blindness or even amputation of the limbs. This is the time to assess the state of the physique, body weight, and lifestyle and visualize what life will be like once the disease strikes. They should imagine the restrictions and the complications that might occur, from blindness to amputation. How much might they have to pay for the rest of their lives in return for short periods of indulgence? It is time to focus on what is important.

Can We Prevent Diabetes?

Prevention of type 1 diabetes is not easy because the roots of the illness are ingrained in a person's genetic makeup. However, efforts are being made in this direction.

The DPP has been designed to initiate research and define measures to deal with this major health problem. Two major primary prevention trials—in collaboration with the National Institute of Diabetes and Digestive and Kidney Diseases (NIDDK) and the NIH, and with the help of private sectors—were conducted in the late 1990s, and the work is in progress. The first trial, Diabetes Prevention Trial of Type 1 (DPT-1), is designed to study the possibility of preventing or delaying the onset of type 1 diabetes. In a number of screening centers, relatives of patients suffering from type 1 diabetes will be investigated for immunological markers and antibodies involved in the immune destruction of beta cells of the pancreas. If antibodies and beta cell damage is found, the individuals may be put on insulin injections or oral capsules of insulin.

The second prevention trial is the DPP. This national study is designed to seek individuals at high risk and prevent or delay the development of type 2 diabetes through drugs, diet, and exercise. Research concerning genetic, metabolic, and behavioral risk factors is reviewed and integrated into a comprehensive model of causation, and preventive measures are proposed. The landmark research and findings in a study trial of people with IGT demonstrated that lifestyle intervention and medicine can reduce the risk of developing type 2 diabetes. Dr. Sherwin, professor of medicine at Yale University and former president of the ADA, said it was worthwhile to detect IGT by screening people in an effort to stave off an epidemic of diabetes, which will cost a fortune later on.[98] The results of the trial translated to a 58 percent reduction in diabetes risk with lifestyle intervention as compared to 31 percent with medicine.[99]

Risk factors such as being overweight and a sedentary lifestyle are potentially reversible. "Lifestyle intervention was significantly better than medicine, no question about it," noted Dr. Nathan, professor of medicine at Harvard University.[100] Lifestyle intervention works across all age, race, and gender groups but is more effective in older people.

The risk factors are reversible and effective in curbing the incidence of diabetes in high-risk individuals. As noted by Anne Maclennan in the *New England Journal of Medicine*, a 7 percent weight loss and 150 minutes of physical activity per week reduced the incidence by 58 percent as compared to medicine, where the decrease in incidence was 31 percent.[101]

A points-based system has been formulated for computing an individual's risk of developing diabetes and cardiovascular disease based on data collected by the San Antonio Heart Study. Kenneth L. Williams presented the model at the annual scientific session of the ADA.[102] For more details please refer to the article "Trends in the Prevalence of the Metabolic Syndrome and Its Impact on Cardiovascular Disease Incidence—The San Antonio Heart Study" by

Carlos Lorenzo, MD; Ken Williams, MS; Kelly J. Hunt, PhD; and Steven M. Haffner, MD *Diabetes Care*, 29:625–630, 2006).

Table 13.1: Assessing Risk of Diabetes

Risk Factors	Percentage
1. Age	
35 to 44 years	5%
45 to 54 years	5%
55 and above	10%
2. Family history of diabetes	20%
3. Fasting blood sugar of 110 mg/dL or more	10%

4. Systolic blood pressure of 160 mm/ Hg or more or diastolic blood pressure of 90 mm Hg or more	10%
5. HDL cholesterol of 35 mg/dL or less	10%
6. Triglycerides of 150 mg/dL	10%
7. Overweight for height	15%
8. High-risk ethnic group	15%

The higher the percentages as calculated from the above table, the higher the risk of developing diabetes.

Obesity Is a Prime Cause of Disease

The NIDDK has conducted research on Pima Indians in Arizona for the past thirty years. This research has helped scientists prove that obesity is a major risk factor in the development of diabetes. Fifty percent of adult Pima Indians are diabetic, and 95 percent of these are overweight. Before gaining weight these individuals were shown to have lower metabolic rates compared to nondiabetic adults of similar weights. Slower metabolic rates and high intakes of fats, combined with greater tendencies to retain fat, are responsible for the high incidence of obesity among the Pima Indians.

Researchers used the "thrifty gene" theory proposed in 1962 by geneticist James Neel to explain the epidemic.[103] James Neel, a professor of human genetics at the University of Michigan Medical School, proposed the "thrifty gene" hypothesis. The Neel theory is based on population studies of communities that relied on farming, hunting, and fishing for thousands of years. These people faced alternating periods of feast and famine. Neel said that to adapt to these extreme changes in calorie needs, these people developed a thrifty gene that allowed them to store extra food in times of plenty, so they would not starve in times of need. Once they adopted a Western lifestyle (less physical activity, excess intake of fatty food, and access to a constant supply of calories), the gene worked against them, and they continued to store excess fat.

Greater-Risk Categories

Anyone can develop diabetes, but certain individuals are more at risk than others:

- People with positive family histories.
- People who are forty years or older.
- People who are overweight, especially with excess fat in the upper part of the abdomen, chest, neck, and face and a waist-to-hip ratio of more than 0.9 in men and 0.8 in women.
- Women who had diabetes during pregnancy or delivered babies weighing nine pounds or more.
- People with high blood pressure.
- People with high blood lipid levels.
- Children born to diabetic mothers.
- People belonging to high-risk ethnic groups, such as African-Americans, Hispanics, Native Americans, and Asians.
- People with IGT on previous testing.

Such persons can prevent or at least delay the onset of diabetes by losing weight, regulating their diets, drastically reducing their consumption of alcohol, and getting regular exercise. They must have their blood sugar, blood lipid, and blood pressure checked regularly.

Precaution for Risk Category

Just as body weight needs to be checked from time to time to keep a watch on it, so does blood sugar have to be checked from time to time to keep diabetes in check, especially in high-risk individuals.

I recommend all individuals thirty years or older get blood sugar and lipid profiles done regularly. This is to detect diabetes in its insipient (prediabetic) stage. This applies more to individuals at greater risk. As the incidence of diabetes is on the rise, these measures will diminish the morbidity.

Pregnant women who are twenty-five years old or more and with high-risk factors should have glucose testing done as early as possible and then between twenty-four and twenty-eight weeks of gestation.

Some research investigations and preliminary data suggest that a higher intake of omega-3 fatty acids, present in fish, might protect people from developing type 2 diabetes.

Drugs that lower blood lipids (cholesterol, triglycerides, and LDL) also help in decreasing the mortality and morbidity in persons with IGT and those with type 2 diabetes.

CHAPTER 14

Do Not Let Our Children Suffer from Diabetes

Preserve our heritage

Are our children at greater risk of developing diabetes? Are the alarm bells ringing? These questions should haunt the minds of parents, teachers, and administrators.

Type 1 Diabetes in Children

Children with diabetes generally suffer from type 1. Every year about thirteen thousand cases of type 1 diabetes are diagnosed.[104] Researchers have made some progress in determining who is at risk for developing this variant, but scientists have not been able to unravel what triggers its onset. It is believed to be a combination of genetic and environmental factors. Efforts are directed toward identifying the external agent that precipitates it. Perhaps a viral infection is responsible for a lethal attack on the insulin-producing cells of the pancreas. Research is directed toward identifying the external source that initiates the autoimmune attack on the beta cells of pancreas, resulting in the almost complete loss of the synthesis of insulin.

Type 2 Diabetes in Children

At present the incidence of type 2 diabetes in children is gaining momentum. Type 2 diabetes is linked to obesity and insulin resistance, and it affects children, teens, and adults. Detecting type 2 diabetes in children can be difficult because children may have mild or no symptoms, and unless blood tests are performed a diagnosis cannot be established. According to statistics published by CDC, type 2 diabetes in children and adolescents in North America is generally found in those between sixteen and nineteen years of age. All ethnic groups suffer, but American Indian youth have the highest prevalence.

Obesity and Diabetes

These children in the United States are obese and insulin resistant, and they have strong family histories of diabetes. Children who lost 5 percent of their body weight reduced their risk of the disease by 61 percent.

The rate of obesity among children has increased dramatically over the past two decades, along with high blood pressure, high blood cholesterol, and diabetes.

According to a recent survey by the CDC, nearly 14 percent of students are overweight in the state of Arkansas, and about 15 percent of American children are overweight. Overweight children may develop chronic diseases that will affect them for life, including type 2 diabetes; this is a growing problem caused by excessive weight and inactivity.[105]

Table 14.1: Percentage of Overweight Students

State	Percent overweight
Texas	14.2
Mississippi	14
North Carolina	12.9
Missouri	12.8

Source: Youth Risk Behavior Survey, 2001[106]

The Responsibilities of Parents

In some homes the morning starts with soda, and the day ends with soda, when it should start with a glass of clean, clear water and end with more water. The parents go to fast-food restaurants, buy hamburgers, come home, and eat sitting in front of the TV. This is the worst thing they can do to their children.

Children are innocent, and they do not know what is right for them. The parents are responsible for teaching their children healthy eating habits. It is sad that the hands that groom, feed, nurture, and protect children are also responsible for showing them the paths of indulgence and sickness.

Precautions during Childhood

Children present unique opportunities for studying preventive maneuvers. Avoiding initial excess weight gain can prevent obesity. With secondary prevention (stopping further gain while the child grows), weight is adjusted naturally. Understanding the origin of obesity is important because it helps parents formulate healthy strategies. It has been found that children predisposed to type 2 diabetes generally have low birth weights and are thin in infancy. They tend to gain weight rapidly in early childhood and become obese in adolescence. It has been reported that even a mild increase in BMI in childhood increases the risk of diabetes.

The association of adult obesity and its complications with birth weight, rebound of the BMI, and being overweight during adolescence shows that these periods may prove critical for the prevention of early overweight and its effect on adult disease, as reported Dr. William Dietz of the CDC. Dr. Dietz is the director of nutrition and physical activity at the CDC in Atlanta. His research is based on childhood obesity.[107]

If a generation of children is diabetic, the cost in terms of health care and lost working hours will run into the billions.

Concerns about childhood obesity necessitate a better understanding of eating habits. An eight-year study conducted at the University of Tennessee has shown that food habits developed in the first two years of life influence habits later in life. The first two years are critical in ensuring healthy food choices, adequate nutrition, and the right amount of calories.

Healthy eating habits can be ensured by following a few simple tips:
- Sodas are rich in nonnutritive calories and put an extra calorie load on the body. They should be avoided.
- Parents should give children three healthy meals and only healthy snacks, such as peanuts or almonds,

between meals. They should not force children to eat unless the children are hungry. When a body needs food, it gives signals, such as emptiness in the pit of the stomach.

- Avoid excess candy and desserts.
- Because children spend lot of time in school, schools should create policies that support physical activity.
- Expose toddlers and children to healthy food choices. Developing the habit of eating generous amounts of fruits and vegetables early in life enhances the chances of their eating them later in life.[108]

The number of older infants and toddlers who are not consuming vegetables is striking. Among children nine to eleven months old, some eat no separate serving of vegetables in a day, and among toddlers older than twelve months, quite a few do not eat vegetables. Healthy diets include many types of foods and have plenty of grain products, fruits, and vegetables, as stated by Vincent Iasnnelli, MD.[109]

It has been shown that eating different-colored fruits and vegetables provides phytonutrients (plant nutrients), which have health benefits.

CHAPTER 15

Managing Diabetes: Diet and Exercise

The good physician treats the disease, the great physician
the patient who has the disease.
-William Osler

This chapter discusses the management of diabetes, particularly the care of the feet and general hygiene. The second section discusses types of exercises (yogic, aerobic, and anaerobic) and the benefits of each. The amount of exercise and calories burned are tabulated. The last part discusses ideal body weight, knowing when weight should be reduced, calorie intake, the nutrient values of foods, and balanced food plans.[110,111,112]

The environment exposes and reveals what we inherit. How much of the environment can be handled depends, to a large extent, on our activities.

I am reminded of a story from the ancient Indian epic *Mahabharata. Karma* means "deed" or "action," and *bhoomi* means "land." The *Mahabharata* epitomizes this philosophy and immortalizes it through an engrossing narration of events: the clash of ambitions, spiraling greed, and a chain of deception and gambles. It culminates in a bloody battle on the fields of Kurakshetra. The Lord's incarnation, Krishna, unveils the essence of man's existence, his spiritual nature, the ethos of religious philosophy, and the laws of karma to his wavering warrior disciple, Arjuna.

As the story unfolds, the ruling monarch and the uncle of the Pandavs split the kingdom of Hastinapur, which rightly belonged to the Pandavs. While the flourishing, bountiful chunk was given to the monarch's eldest son, a small piece of barren land was given to the Pandavs.

When the despairing Pandavs turned to Lord Krishna, they were told, "This is your karma bhoomi," meaning, "From this land you carve out your destiny with your deeds."

Your body is akin to your bhoomi, and how well you look after your health, which is your karma, will decide its destiny.

Diabetes Is Mainly a Self-Managed Condition

Management of type 1 diabetes is different from treatment of type 2. Although the goal is to achieve normal blood glucose levels in all types of diabetes, other factors greatly modify treatment. Age, sex, working circumstances, overall health status, and lifestyle influence the management objectives. Requirements in young children differ from those in elderly adults. Similarly the demands for middle-aged and working women are different because pregnancy and menstrual cycles pose their own challenges. When to eat, how much to eat, the types of food, the doses of medicine, and the amounts and types of exercise vary from person to person, so treatment goals must be tailored to individual demands.

Regimes and Treatments of Individual Demands
The treatment of diabetes requires management of multiple aspects. For patients and their relatives, diabetes management becomes a team effort that takes a multidisciplinary approach.

Acute and chronic hazards of the disease should be recognized and treated early to prevent irreversible damage.

An overenthusiastic approach in the treatment regime and an attempt to achieve normal blood glucose levels may cause hypoglycemia, especially when the patient is taking insulin. Such episodes occur more often in type 1 diabetes because the patients are totally dependent on insulin for managing their disease.

Hypoglycemia
This is a common, dangerous condition in diabetes. (For more see page 117.)

Care of the Feet
The care of the feet cannot be overemphasized because neglect can cause morbidity and even mortality. The feet should be washed daily with soap and water. They should be dried, especially between the toes, and not rubbed too vigorously to avoid cracking the delicate skin. After drying, patients should rub vegetable oil or moisturizer on the feet to prevent cracks and dryness. They should not walk barefoot. Their shoes should never be tight; they should be wide and have low heels and must be well fitting, comfortable, and preferably made of leather. The feet should be inspected daily for cuts or abrasions, and if there are any they should be treated immediately. Any red or blue patches should be given immediate attention. Patients should not cut any corns. They should cut the toenails straight and avoid

cutting the corners. If the feet tend to remain moist and might develop fungal infections, a dusting powder should be used.

Many diabetic patients have cold feet due to vascular and circulatory disturbances (cold constricts the blood vessels). In such situations they can wear warm stockings. They should avoid socks with tight elastic bands because these compress the vessels and further impair circulation.

Patients should avoid tobacco in any form because it contracts the blood vessels and decreases circulation. Hot water pads and heat should be avoided because they tend to burn delicate skin. If an ulcer develops, it should be treated under medical supervision. If neglected an ulcer can become infected, leading to a nonhealing wound, which may result in amputation. The ulcerated area should be rested and kept elevated and free of pressure. A number of ointments that promote healing are available. These should be used after medical consultation.

Diet Management

> While we need so little to survive, we need so much to appease our appetites.
>
> —Rita Malik

No doubt there were those who thought Hippocrates, the father of modern medicine, was behind the times when he said, "Let food be your medicine and medicine be your food." He was a visionary who thought, ahead of his time, that diet management was the key to diabetes control. Thomas Edison, the inventing visionary, said the doctor of the future would give no medicine but would help patients through diet and learning the causes of disease.

Meal planning is crucial in controlling diabetes. A well-balanced, nutritious diet is required. The diet must be tailored to the person's metabolic rate and lifestyle requirements. In obese patients with type 2 diabetes, the focus is on weight reduction. Such patients must reduce their intake of carbohydrates and fats. Portions of carbohydrates can be replaced with monounsaturated fats, such as olive oil and rapeseed oil (canola). This also applies to patients in whom it is difficult to get good glycemic control, especially those with type 1 diabetes who are on insulin therapy.

For all people with diabetes, total cholesterol content should not exceed 300 mg per day. The total protein content should constitute 10 to 20 percent of daily calorie intake; monounsaturated fats should be about 10 percent, and polyunsaturated should be another 10 percent. Saturated fats are to be discouraged for all individuals.

Losing weight is part of treating type 2 diabetes. Losing weight means eating less, and eating less means fewer calories. Fat is the most concentrated form of calories, so the best way to lose weight is to cut down on fats, especially saturated fats.

Body Weight

An ideal body weight is the first prerequisite for good health, but for a diabetic it is essential.

If type 2 diabetes is associated with obesity, the first line of management is weight reduction. This and diet control may be sufficient to manage the condition.

A healthy body weight helps to prevent IGT from progressing to type 2 diabetes. It also helps reverse the failure to respond to drugs. It reduces blood pressure, improves the lipid profile, and reduces the risk of death from complications. In determining calorie needs, it is necessary to know the person's ideal body weight. The optimal weight for men and women for three body frame sizes are given below.

For Men between Twenty-Five and Fifty-Nine Years (Weight in Pounds)

5' 2"	128–150
5' 3"	130–153
5' 4"	132–156
5' 5"	134–160
5' 6"	136–164
5' 7"	138–172
5' 8"	140–176
5' 9"	142–180
5' 10'	144–180
5' 11"	146–184
6' 0"	149–188
6' 1"	152–192
6' 2"	155–197
6' 3"	158–202
6' 4"	162–202

For Women between Twenty-Five and Fifty Years (Weight in Pounds)

4' 10"	102–132
4' 11"	103–134
5' 0"	104–137
5' 1"	106–140
5' 2"	108–143
5' 3"	111–147
5' 4"	114–151
5' 5"	117–155
5' 6"	120–159
5' 7"	123–163
5' 8"	126–167
5' 9"	129–170
5' 10"	132–173
5' 11"	135–176
6' 0"	138–179

A simple formula to calculate ideal body weight is as follows:
- Men: 50 kg for the first five feet of height plus 2.3 kg for each additional inch
- Women: 45.5 kg for the first five feet of height plus 2.3 kg for each additional inch

An obese person weighs 20 percent more than the ideal body weight.

Calorie Requirements

The total calorie content eaten daily varies from person to person depending on age, sex, height, metabolic rate, and lifestyle.

The minimum daily requirement is 10 calories per pound of ideal body weight. This means if the person's ideal weight is 150 pounds, the basic requirement is 1,500 calories per day. Additional calories are added depending on the degree of activity. For a person leading a sedentary life, add 10 percent of the basal calorie requirement; for a person with a moderate degree of activity, add 20 percent; and for a person with an active life, 40 percent or more is needed.

For example, a person with an ideal body weight of 150 pounds and leading a moderately active life needs 1,500 calories plus 20 percent of 1,500 (300 calories), totaling 1,800 calories. A person about fifty years of age, doing light to moderate activity, requires an additional 300 calories per day. A young person with a vigorous daily routine needs 1,000 or more calories in addition to the basic recommended intake (2,500 to 3,000 calories per day). A diabetic woman who is pregnant or lactating needs an additional 1,000 calories or more.

When trying to lose weight, the number of calories consumed must correspondingly decrease. Body weight is determined by the number of calories eaten minus the number of calories burned by activity.

One gram of protein and one gram of carbohydrate yield four calories, whereas one gram of alcohol gives seven calories and one gram of fat gives nine calories.

After determining the calorie intake requirement, the meals of the day can be planned.

Dietary fibers should constitute an important portion of the daily food intake. There are two types of fibers: soluble and insoluble.

The insoluble fibers are cellulose and hemicellulose. These are found in bran and green, leafy vegetables, such as spinach, mustard leaves, cabbage, and lettuce. As these are not absorbed from the intestinal tract, they help form the bulk of the waste that collects in the large intestine, which is necessary for optimal intestinal motility (motion). Intestinal motility is required for healthy colonic functions and prevents the stagnation of food residue in the gut. This minimizes the contact of harmful ingredients (such as carcinogens) with the wall of colon, and it reduces the absorption of articles in the diet such as cholesterol.

The soluble fibers, which include gums and pectins, are found in oatmeal, apples, and beans. These retard the rates of absorption of nutrients, thereby diminishing a rapid rise of blood sugar levels at meals. They also lower LDL cholesterol in the blood and increase HDL cholesterol. As the saying goes, an apple a day keeps the doctor away.

A Vegetarian Diet Is Better than a Nonvegetarian Diet

A vegetarian diet obtained from plants—cereals, lentils, beans, fruits, and vegetables—is rich in fiber content. These foods contain complex carbohydrates and have polyunsaturated and monounsaturated fats. A nonvegetarian diet obtained from animals—red meat, poultry, milk, and milk products—contains a high content of saturated fats, no fiber, and simple sugars that are rapidly absorbed and raise blood glucose levels. A vegetarian diet including thirty to forty grams of fiber per day is highly recommended for diabetic patients.

Water

A lot is written about the food we eat, and types of food and dietary requirements are frequently discussed. Food is important, but water is no less important. An adequate amount of water must be consumed each day. This is important for optimal kidney and bowel functions. It is also required for fully hydrated, healthy skin, which excretes sweat along with body waste and helps maintain body temperature.

The air we breathe and the water we drink are the two most important elements required for well-being. Pure, clean water is essential for healthy living. Drinking bottled water is a possible alternative, but one has to be sure of the source because bottled water is often repackaged from a pipeline supply. Drinking filtered water is an option, especially in third world countries where drinking water supplied by pipelines is of questionable purity. Filtered water is more reliable.

There are many types of water filters that can be installed in homes. If obtained from standard manufacturers, and if regularly serviced, most of them are good enough. Most use carbon-block filtration, which removes organic chemicals, and other mechanisms that are effective against inorganic pollutants like lead and nitrates.

A water filtration method developed in Japan forms "microwater." The water is filtered, and the water molecules are made smaller. A small electrical charge is injected into the water, and this separates it into two types: acidic and alkaline. Acidic water is used for external and topical purposes, and alkaline water is used for drinking.

According to Dr. Hayashi, one of Japan's foremost microwater researchers, the alkaline water is a powerful antioxidant similar to vitamins A, C, and E. Like other antioxidants it destroys harmful chemicals liberated in the body during metabolism. Because the water molecule is smaller, it can penetrate the cells and tissues more effectively, enabling it to deliver nutrients to the cells and remove waste better. According to Hayashi those who have been drinking microwater every day for several months have shown improvement in their diabetes, blood pressure, allergies, obesity, osteoporosis, and other irregularities. Some firms in California are producing microwater units that can be easily installed in homes. The alkaline water tastes like mountain spring water.

For more details on microwater, refer to *The Definitive Guide to Cancer* by W. John Diamond, MD, and W. Lee Cowden, MD, with Burton Goldberg.

Proteins

Proteins constitute an important and essential ingredient in the diet. On average a man requires a minimum of fifty grams and a woman a minimum of forty grams of protein per day. Growing children and pregnant and lactating mothers require an extra fifteen to twenty grams per day (not to exceed 15 percent of total calorie intake). Persons doing active physical labor do not need extra protein if their intakes of carbohydrate and fat are adequate.

Proteins are essential for the growth and maintenance of tissues because they constitute an integral part of the tissues, especially muscles. Proteins are also required for the synthesis of hormones and enzymes. Amino acids are the building blocks of proteins, and most of these can be synthesized in the body when required. About nine essential amino acids cannot be prepared by the body and need to be consumed in our food. Proteins obtained from animal sources, such as poultry, fish, and dairy products, are rich in essential amino acids whereas proteins obtained from plant sources lack one or more essential amino acids.

It is recommended that at least 50 percent of a person's protein intake should come from animal sources to ensure an adequate supply of essential amino acids.

With wear and tear of the tissues, amino acids are lost and need to be replenished. Among the amino acids, proline and lysine are important building blocks of collagen fiber, which is needed to preserve the stability of blood vessel walls. The plant proteins present in cereals, beans, and lentils are considered good sources of amino acids. The proteins found in soybeans_are highly concentrated. Soybeans also contain phytoestrogen and isoflavones, which are said to decrease the incidence of prostate cancer in men and breast cancer in women. Other beans also contain phytoestrogen, and these help in reducing menopausal symptoms.

An egg yolk has more than 200 mg of cholesterol and is considered unhealthy. Fish is regarded among the best forms of proteins from animal sources; besides proteins it contains oils rich in vitamins and omega-3 fatty acids, which are good for the heart. Omega-3 fatty acids are long-chain polyunsaturated fatty acids that help increase the HDL cholesterol level in blood, which is protective in nature. The Eskimos, living in the circumpolar region extending from Alaska, Canada, and Siberia to Greenland, consume lot of fat in the form of fish oils but remain at lower risk for cancer and heart disease. Mackerel, sardines, and herring are considered better sources of omega-3 fatty acids, which have three double bonds.

Too much protein is bad for the health. Excess protein is lost in urine, thereby overloading the kidneys. The amino acids remove calcium from the bones when they are excreted, and this leads to osteoporosis.

Carbohydrates

Carbohydrates are required to provide energy in the body and should be about 55 to 65 percent of a person's calorie intake. Carbohydrates are classified as simple (sugars) and complex (starches).

A diabetic patient should avoid sugars. Not only do they constitute a concentrated form of calories, but they lack nutrients, rapidly raise blood glucose levels, and cause tooth decay.

Complex carbohydrates found in cereals, lentils, legumes, and beans are highly recommended because they are rich in fiber and nutrients. Cereals include wheat, oat, barley, and rice, and they need to be eaten in the whole (not refined) form, otherwise the fiber content is lost. Oats are beneficial because they lower LDL cholesterol and raise HDL cholesterol. Barley is considered even better in this respect.

Artificial Sweeteners

There are natural sugars (sucrose or cane sugar) and artificial sweeteners. Sugars have no nutritive value and only add calories. Their continuous use increases the desire for sweets. Foods with high sugar contents impair glucose control and should be eaten sparingly, and the desire for sweets should be mitigated at all costs.

Artificial sweeteners, such as saccharin and Sunett®, have no calorie value. Aspartame has very little or insignificant calorie content.[113]

The Federal Drug Administration (FDA) has approved the following five artificial sweeteners for the market:
1. Aspartame (NutraSweet or Equal)
2. Acesulfame potassium (Sunett®)
3. D-tagatose (Sugaree)
4. Sucralose (Splenda®)

5. Saccharin (Sweet'N Low). This compound was introduced in 1879, and it is three hundred times sweeter
   than sugar.

An herbal sweetener called stevia has been used by South
American natives for many centuries and in Japan since the
mid-1970s.

Natural sweeteners, such as sorbitol and fructose, have
become popular as sweetening agents. These may cause diarrhea, and, taken in high doses, they tend to raise LDL cholesterol. When eaten in fruits and in small amounts, they are not
harmful, but a diabetic should exercise restraint and eat them
in moderation.

The FDA gave approval to a nonnutritive sweetener, sucralose,
on August 12, 1999. Sucralose is derived from table sugar and
used in food products. It is believed to be six hundred times as
sweet as sugar.

Fatty Alarm

Fats are the richest and most concentrated source of energy.
They are tasty and give a sense of satiety, so people tend to consume more fats in their diets. In the body fats help produce
energy.

Fats eaten in excess are stored in fat depots and cause obesity, with all the harmful consequences. Calories that are not
burned are also stored in the form of fat. Nature created fat as
a food reserve in the body, but if too much is stored, the result
is dangerous.

No more than thirty-five grams of fats should be consumed per day, and the total calorie intake in the form of fats should not exceed 20 percent. If the calorie requirement is high, the amount of fat intake may be increased to forty-five grams.

Fats fall into two categories: cholesterol and fatty acids (with their derivative, triglycerides). Cholesterol is present as a structural component of the cell membrane. The body can easily synthesize it, and we do not require cholesterol from an external source. If we consume cholesterol, we raise the cholesterol level in the blood, which is not good for the heart.

Fatty acids are saturated, monounsaturated, or polyunsaturated.

Saturated Fatty Acids

Saturated fatty acids are associated with increased incidence of heart attacks, and it is strongly recommended that people avoid this type of fats. Foods from animal sources, such as beef, meat, pork, eggs, and chicken, are rich in saturated fatty acids, and fats present in dairy products are of the same type.

Unsaturated Fatty Acids

It is recommended that diets include the unsaturated fatty acids (preferably monounsaturated) found in olive oil, canola oil, avocados, and complex carbohydrates. They are also found in peanuts, pistachios, and cashews.

A polyunsaturated fatty acid called linoleic acid (found in corn, peanuts, walnuts, cottonseed oil, soybeans, and many plant oils) is an essential nutrient and should be present in our food because we cannot synthesize it. A deficiency of it causes hair loss and impaired wound healing. Other essential fatty acids include linoleic acid (found in lin-seed oil) and arachidonic acid. These are found along with linoleic acid. These compounds constitute the structural integrity of the cells, and they occur in high concentrations in the reproductive organs. The deficiency of these essential fatty acids in experimental rats has been shown to cause skin disorders and reproductive deficiency.

At room temperature saturated fats are solid, and unsaturated fats are fluid.

Vitamins

Vitamins, minerals, and trace metals constitute important ingredients that cells require to perform their metabolic functions and generate bioenergy. Each cell in the body needs energy for optimum functioning.

Vitamins, beta-carotene, lysine, proline, bioflavonoids, carnitine, and coenzyme Q10[114,115,116] are useful in the prevention of diabetes, hypertension, and atherosclerosis.

Dr. Linus Pauling, a two-time Nobel laureate, did extensive work in nutritional research and cellular medicine. He advocated that health is determined at the cellular level. Cells require vitamins and other essential nutrients to perform millions of chemical reactions, and the deficiency of these ingredients will eventually lead to the malfunction of the cells and disease. The organs and systems that work the hardest undergo the most wear and tear and bear a greater brunt of the deficiency.

Vitamins are a group of organic compounds that constitute essential portions of our dietary requirements because the body cannot synthesize these molecules. They are divided into water-soluble and fat-soluble compounds.

Water-soluble vitamins include C and B, and the fat-soluble vitamins are A, D, E, and K. Foods containing these nutrients have been used as therapy for thousands of years. Ancient Egyptians ate the livers of roosters to cure night blindness because they were rich in vitamin A. They also ate sea sponges, a natural source of iodine, to treat goiter.

Too much of anything is bad, and excess vitamins and minerals in the form of supplements should be discouraged unless prescribed by a doctor. Fat-soluble vitamins, when taken in excess, are stored in the fat depots in the body while excess water-soluble vitamins are lost in urine.

Vitamins and minerals are crucial to good health. They do not release energy, but some of them form part of the enzymes that release energy from fats and carbohydrates. Every cell requires minerals and vitamins in different proportions and for different purposes (for example, bones and teeth need calcium the most).

Vitamin A

Vitamin A is required for maintenance of the skin and the linings of the oral cavity, stomach, intestine, and food pipe. It also helps in the growth of bone and teeth, and deficiency of it can produce blindness in children. It is needed for healthy skin and strong bones, teeth, and eyes. It is found in carrots; green, leafy vegetables, such as spinach; broccoli; mangoes; apricots; watermelon; cantaloupe; sweet potatoes; and tuna. The recommended amount of vitamin A is 5,000 IUs (international units) per day.

Vitamin B1 (Thiamine)

This vitamin is essential for a healthy nervous system and carbohydrate metabolism. It functions as a cofactor for pyrophosphate, which acts as a catalyst in carbohydrate metabolism to produce energy bonds required by the cells. Wheat, rice bran, peanuts, legumes, oatmeal, oranges, watermelon, and eggs contain it. The daily requirement is 1.5 mg.

Vitamin B2 (Riboflavin)

This vitamin benefits fat, protein, and carbohydrate metabolism and functions as a cofactor for adenine dinucleotide, which is one of the most important carrier molecules of high-energy bonds in the cells. It is available in dairy products, fish, cereals, mushrooms, turnips, broccoli, and turkey. The daily need is 1.7 mg.

Vitamin B3 (Niacin)

This vitamin is needed for the metabolism of fat, protein, and starches; the optimal utilization of oxygen by the cells; and the functional physiology of the nervous system. It is an essential component of nicotinamide adenine dinucleotide, an important carrier of high-energy bonds in the power plants of the cells. It is found in peanut butter, legumes, soybeans, whole-grain cereals, broccoli, meat, poultry, and fish. The daily requirement is 20 mg.

Vitamin B5 (Pantothenic Acid)

This is used in fat, protein, and carbohydrate metabolism. It is a cofactor in acetyl coenzyme A, a key molecule in the production of high-energy bonds. It is found in fish, whole-grain cereals, avocados, peanuts, cashews, lentils, soybeans, and eggs. The daily need is 10 mg.

Vitamin B6 (Pyridoxine)

This vitamin is required for protein metabolism for normal growth and is essential for strong immunity. It is also needed for the production of red blood cells, which transport oxygen in the circulation. It is present in fish, soybeans, bananas, cauliflower, potatoes, green peppers, spinach, raisins, and chicken. An intake of 2 mg each day is sufficient.

Vitamin B12

This vitamin is required for red blood cell formation, optimal function of the nervous system, and new tissue growth. It is found in salmon, eggs, cheese, tuna, crab, oysters, swordfish, and mussels. The daily need is 6 mcg (micrograms).

Folic acid and vitamins B6 and B12 are required for the synthesis of red blood cells, which carry oxygen in the blood. Life is not possible without oxygen, so it is imperative to take adequate amounts of these vitamins.

Folic acid

This is used in the formation of red blood cells and for tissue growth and repair. It is found in tuna, poultry, wheat, mushrooms, bananas, strawberries, cantaloupe, and oranges. The daily need is 0.4 mg.

Biotin

This vitamin benefits fat, protein, and carbohydrate metabolism. Natural sources are eggs, nuts (especially peanuts), oatmeal, wheat germ, legumes, and cauliflower. The daily requirement is 0.3 mg; higher doses may be given to people with diabetes.

Vitamin C

This vitamin is required in the growth and maintenance of the ground substance of the tissues of the body. It is required for the production of collagen fibers (elastic fibers and connective tissue molecules that bind tissues and cells together). Just as a building can collapse without cement, the cells lose their format without collagen, as is seen in scurvy. This vitamin is needed for the continuous repair and regeneration of tissues that are lost in the wear and tear of cells. Vitamin C is required for healing tiny abrasions that occur in the linings of blood vessels and other hollow structures. The vessel wall abrasions hold special significance because they predispose a person to atherosclerosis.

Vitamin C is also required by the energy carrier's molecules in the cells, and it is a strong antioxidant. It is found in rich concentration in citrus fruits such as oranges and grapefruit; in vegetables such as cabbage, broccoli, and tomatoes; and in fruits such as raspberries and strawberries. The daily requirement is 60 mg, but 500 to 1,000 mg is recommended for healing conditions. Some authorities recommend up to 2,000 mg for people with diabetes.

Vitamin D

This vitamin is needed for the metabolism of calcium and the growth and maintenance of bones and teeth. It is found in milk and milk products, tuna, salmon, cereals, and eggs. Without an adequate amount of vitamin D, growth is retarded, and the bones become weak and malformed. The daily requirement is 400 IU.

Vitamin E

This vitamin is a strong antioxidant, and it protects cells from damage. It is also believed to keep the blood thin and less sticky. It is found in peanuts, wheat germ, mangoes, blackberry, broccoli, spinach, and apples. The daily need is 30 IU.

Vitamin K

This vitamin is required for the blood to clot. It is present in spinach, broccoli, brussels sprouts, cabbage, parsley, carrots, tomatoes, and dairy products. The daily requirement is 6 mcg.

Antioxidants: The Protective Shield

Antioxidants are substances that neutralize the effects of free oxygen radicals and superoxides that are liberated during metabolic activity (more so during infection and inflammation). The free oxygen radicals and superoxides are increased by the consumption of alcohol and cured meat. Herbicides, asbestos, chemotherapeutic drugs (used in cancer treatment), and exposure to ultraviolet rays, X-rays, and car exhaust also induce the production of these radicals. Food preservatives, coloring, frying, and barbecuing foods have similar effects.

Superoxides and free oxygen radicals are highly reactive molecules that damage cells. Antioxidants prevent their action.

These radicals induce degeneration in the tissues and enhance the aging process. They also act on the chromosomal matter of cells and induce cancer formation. A prerequisite for the deposition of LDL cholesterol in the walls of blood vessels is the oxidation of LDL by these radicals, which leads to atherosclerosis. Free radicals can damage the pancreas, producing diabetes, and act on the lenses of the eyes, causing cataract.

These radicals also compromise the immune system. The levels of these chemicals are higher in diabetics, making them vulnerable to damage by oxygen radicals.

Today the front line in treating diabetes and other diseases of old age, such as cancer and heart disease, is high doses of antioxidants. Vitamins A, E, and C are good antioxidants. Phytochemicals are powerful antioxidants present in fruits and leafy green vegetables, such as cabbage; broccoli; carrots; tomatoes; citrus fruits; ginger; and garlic. Soy and cereals also have antioxidants, as do beverages such as tea and coffee, nuts such as peanuts, fish, and curd containing acidophilus.

Phytochemicals have strong anticancer activity; they retard tumor growth and are powerful inhibitors of breast, colon, and prostate cancer. They block the absorption of cholesterol from the gut, lower the level of cholesterol in the blood, and prevent the clogging of blood vessels, thereby reducing the incidence of heart disease and hypertension.

Green tea is an age-old panacea. The Chinese discovered it thousands of years ago, and they found that it helped ward off infections and made drinkers feel energetic. Health experts now agree that green tea, which is full of antiaging vitamins, lowers cholesterol, improves circulation, and protects against skin cancer and arthritis.

Herbal teas containing rosemary, oregano, basil, peppermint, and turmeric also act as antioxidants and have been found useful in treating diabetes and arthritis.

Beta-carotene is called provitamin A. It is an important fat-soluble antioxidant that decreases the risk of blood clots.

Minerals such as iron, copper, zinc, selenium, magnesium, and chromium also act as antioxidants.

Zinc is found in seafood, legumes, nuts, and dairy products. A diabetic patient requires about 30 mg per day.

Magnesium is found in nuts, wheat germ, seafood, broccoli, and bananas. An average of 300 mg per day is needed. The routine evaluation of serum magnesium levels is necessary because a deficiency of this element can cause insulin resistance, carbohydrate intolerance, and hypertension.

Manganese is an important cofactor in the key enzymes of glucose metabolism.

A daily dosage of 30 mg is recommended.

Selenium is found in whole grains, dairy products, fish, mushrooms, and nuts. About 200 mg are needed per day.

Chromium

Chromium is required for the optimum use of glucose and insulin. It is found in whole grains, broccoli, black pepper, oranges, grapes, and cheese. A daily dose of 300 mg is required.

Recent studies have shown significant beneficial effects of chromium. Administration of this element has shown improvement in both mild glucose intolerance and frank diabetes. It improved lipid variables in type 2 diabetes in a study carried out in the Chinese population. Women with gestational diabetes were also seen to benefit from chromium intake.[117,118] Recent research has shown that steroid therapy increases the loss of chromium, and replacement of this mineral can reverse steroid-induced diabetes.[119] Ongoing research in this field will be informative.

Garlic and onion have significant blood sugar lowering actions due to sulfur-containing compounds (e.g., allyl propyl disulphide, present in onions, and diallyl disulfide oxide, present in garlic). Onions, especially their skins, contain a compound called quercetin, which helps to decrease eye problems associated with diabetes.

Coenzyme Q10

This enzyme is vital in the use of oxygen and the healthy sustenance of cells.[120] The secretion of this enzyme, like many others, slows down as age advances, and the body suffers from its deficiency. This compound is marketed as tablets, and the dose prescribed is 60 mg per day.

Soy Foods

Soy foods have become popular and are known as cholesterol killers because of their effects on blood cholesterol. In several studies researchers found a correlation between the intake of soy foods and blood cholesterol. It was found that when people with high cholesterol levels replaced animal protein in their diet with soy protein, their levels of total cholesterol, triglycerides, and LDL cholesterol decreased while the level of HDL cholesterol increased. Scientists noted that in countries like China and Japan, where soy foods are a staple in the diet, the incidences of heart attacks and osteoporosis are low. The incidences of breast, ovarian, and prostate cancers are much lower compared to the incidence in America.[121]

Soybeans are legumes and, like other beans, contain chemicals known as isoflavones or phytoestrogens. These chemicals (especially one called genistein) are similar to human estrogens but weaker, and when ingested they probably block the action of normal, stronger estrogens by blocking the receptors. Despite research in this field, it is not known what component in soy protein is responsible for lowering blood cholesterol levels or the mechanism by which it operates.

Soybeans are a good source of calcium, copper, magnesium, and many B vitamins. They are also high in fiber content.

It is widely advocated that the regular consumption of soy achieves the following:
1. Decreases fat storage
2. Increases the fat burning rate
3. Increases lean muscle mass
4. Provides energy for activity
5. Lowers blood cholesterol and the risks of heart disease and stroke
6. Serves as a rich source of protein
7. Minimizes insulin fluctuations

Soy has a low glycemic index of eighteen.

The following food supplements are also recommended for people with diabetes.

Alpha Lipoic Acid
This is considered a powerful antioxidant. It improves the effectiveness of other antioxidants, especially vitamins C and E. It may help in the use of insulin, reducing insulin resistance and thereby improving glucose utilization. It repairs nerve damage and helps in treating diabetic neuropathy. Visual improvement

in patients with glaucoma is reported. The recommended daily intake is 100 to 800 mg, and research in its use continues.

Vanadyl Sulfate

This is believed to help in the proper metabolism of glucose. Patients with kidney insufficiency should not take it.

Aloe Vera

This wonder plant has been in use for thousands of years. Its benefits have been described in ancient Indian texts. It contains important ingredients, including vitamins C and E, some essential minerals, and amino acids, and it is a powerful anti-oxidant. It also contains saponins and lignins that bind to toxic waste in the body. It is a potent stimulant for the immune system and helps curb infections and heal wounds, and the extract has been used for treating skin burns. It is an herb with a succulent, juicy interior and a thorny exterior. It has a bitter taste. Some people eat it whole and raw while others eat the succulent interior.

Spices

Spices such as cinnamon, turmeric, clove, coriander, and cumin are believed to help increase response and sensitivity of tissues to the action of insulin.

Diets for Diabetics

A sensible diet for diabetics is based on cereals with lots of fruits and vegetables. People with diabetes should eat a vegetarian diet, eat whole fruits rather than drink fruit juice, eat a moderate amount of dairy products, and drink plenty of plain water rather than soft drinks. It is also advisable to eat homemade meals rather than fast food. They should consider replacing animal proteins with plant proteins because animal food is devoid of fiber.

In ancient India, when Ayurveda was the mode of treatment, doctors prescribed apples to relieve diarrhea. Apples are rich in pectin, a soluble fiber. Fiber regulates intestinal motility and reduces the absorption of cholesterol, thereby decreasing the risk of heart disease and cancer. Green leafy vegetables are rich sources of fiber and minerals. Carrots have beta-carotene, and cranberry juice helps kill bacteria.

Cereals form staple diets all over the world. Pasta is preferred in Italy, chapatis in India, bread in Britain, and tortillas in Mexico. Each preparation is inspiring in its own right. Although they vary in starch content, they all share a low fat content, have a fair amount of protein, and are tremendously satisfying. While wheat remains the main source, other grains such as rice and oatmeal are equally good. The US Department of Agriculture food pyramid recommends that people eat six to eleven servings from the cereal, rice, and pasta group each day.

An adult man with diabetes would include the following each day to consume an average of 1,800 to 2,000 calories:
  1. Six helpings of cereals.
  2. Three helpings of vegetables.
  3. Three helpings of dairy products.
  4. Two helpings of fruits.
  5. Two helpings of meat, fish, or poultry.

Table 15.1: The Equivalents of Various Helpings

One helping of cereal	One piece of bread One small, ready-to-eat tortilla One-half cup of cooked cereal, pasta, rice, puffed cereal, or cornmeal
One helping of vegetables	One cup of leafy vegetables Two-thirds cup of cooked vegetables
One helping of fruit	One medium apple, banana, or orange One-half grapefruit
One helping of dairy products	One-half cup of milk One-half cup of yogurt One-half ounce of cheese
One helping of meat	Two ounces of cooked lean meat, fish, or poultry One egg

It is recommended that people eat no more than two eggs, four ounces of cheese, four ounces of red meat, and eight ounces of poultry per week. They should eat a minimum of three fish meals per week.

It is advisable to eat chicken without the skin, which is rich in saturated fats. Another way to decrease the fat content of poultry and red meat is to boil it before cooking and throw away the water. (Never use this water for soups or other dishes.) Avoid rich sauces; eat clear soups instead of creamy preparations, and eat salads as appetizers rather than fried preparations.

Exercise

Exercise is the key in managing diabetes. It helps burn calories, and it has been found that half an hour of moderate exercise brings the blood glucose level down by nearly 40 mg percent.

The increased metabolic rate induced by activity remains high for some time after the activity ends. The most beneficial effect is the improvement of circulation to every organ of the body. This improved blood supply provides nutrition to the cells and removes waste material. Most important is the improved oxygen supply to the tissues, which helps them to use food better and improves their vitality. Exercise increases the muscle mass of the body, which raises the metabolic rate. It increases the strength of the heart and the circulation in the blood vessels, and it improves the stroke volume, thereby decreasing the incidences of angina and heart attacks.

Exercise helps reduce obesity and therefore the severity of diabetes. For many patients doses of insulin and other antidiabetic drugs are significantly reduced.

A sedentary lifestyle has been linked to 28 percent of deaths caused by chronic diseases.
- Exercise should be encouraged not only because of its beneficial effects on blood pressure, cardiovascular conditions, diabetes, and osteoporosis but also because it improves mood and cures insomnia.
- It is believed that improved circulation to the brain helps secrete hormones that elevate mood, help people

perform better, give them a sense of satisfaction, eliminate worries, and induce sound sleep. It is well known that a laborer sleeps much better than an executive.

- Exercise raises the level of HDL cholesterol, decreases the risk of coronary disease, lowers both systolic and diastolic blood pressure, and decreases the risk of cancer.

- An important factor that is often missed in discussions of exercise is motivation. People often have some excuse or another that prevents them from doing a daily workout. Their lives are hectic swirls; they are too tired; health clubs are not accessible; or something else. None of these reasons should deter them. The greatest motivation for exercise is the knowledge that exercise keeps them agile and healthy. All that is required to feel fit and healthy is to incorporate a little more physical activity in daily routines.

- Even when there is no health club available and life is busy, there is always time for a leisurely walk on a footpath or in a mall. It is not necessary to do high-intensity workouts, especially for people who are old and somewhat disabled. A thirty-minute daily walk has significant health benefits. It decreases blood pressure and blood cholesterol, improves heart function, and reduces the risk of heart disease.

- Strenuous aerobic exercise is good if you are in decent shape and enjoy it, said Dr. Duncan of the Cooper Institute for Aerobics Research in Dallas, but it is not essential. What matters is exercise regularity. If you become a little more active in your daily life, your health improves significantly.[122]

James Rippe, MD, director of the Exercise Physiology and Nutrition Laboratory at the University of Massachusetts Medical Center, asked volunteers to walk on treadmills at slow, medium, and fast speeds. No matter what speed they walked, observed Dr. Rippe, all felt equally less tense and less stressed afterward.[123]

Before you start any exercise program, a complete physical examination is advised, especially for men older than forty and women older than fifty. Your limitations or disabilities, if any, must be taken into consideration before you embark on any exercise schedule.

Yoga or Yogic Exercises

Yoga is the fusion of science and philosophy. Yogic exercises are mild and are performed gradually, without jerks or violent movements. The exercises are designed to improve the microcirculation of the tissues, which is essential for the vitality of the organs. Yogic postures, or asanas, cleanse the body and the soul. By improving microcirculation, toxins are removed from the body.[124]

The word *yoga* means "union," and the yogic postures are believed to unite the body with the mind. This sounds obscure, but the message is a deep, fundamental truth: the supremacy of mind over body. The mind controls the body's functions and channels its energies into productive activity. Yogic exercise allows the release of positive neurotransmitters in the brain that induce healthy activity in the body.

Yoga improves the flexibility of joints, increases muscle strength, relieves stress, removes negative thoughts, stills the mind, and enables you to experience relaxation and tranquility. The key elements of yoga are proper breathing, gentle exercises, and meditation, which heals all ailments.

The breathing exercises are the most important. They improve the total capacity of the lungs, eliminate toxins, improve the oxygen saturation of the blood, and increase oxygen delivery to the tissues. This is vital for burning glucose to obtain energy. Lack of oxygen to the tissues depletes them of energy and causes fatigue. Yoga emphasizes exhalation rather than inhalation, and it teaches you to breathe through the nose.

Some of the easy and important asanas are detailed below. Between the asanas and at the beginnings and ends of yogic exercises, it is important to perform the corpse pose. All asanas are to be performed on the floor. You should be completely at ease, and the environment should be peaceful. The best time to do yoga is early in the morning. It may be done late in the evening, but whatever the time it should be done without rushing.

Corpse Pose

Lie on your back, keeping your arms at your sides at a forty-five degree angle. Your palms should face upward, and your legs should be straight, with your feet in a relaxed position, about twenty inches apart. Close your eyes and relax all the muscles in your body. Remain in this pose for few minutes, and experience total relaxation.

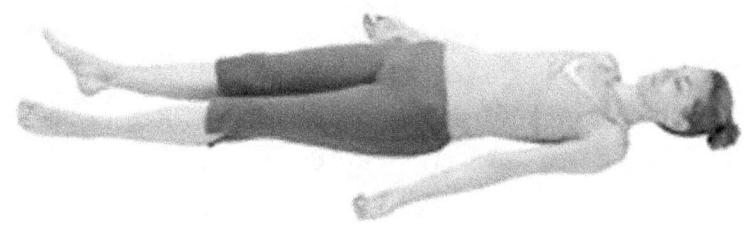

MARTIN SCONDUTO

Corpse pose (*savasna*)[125]

Abdominal Breathing

Lie flat on your back, placing both hands on your abdomen, and inhale deeply. When you feel your abdomen rising, exhale, and feel your abdomen falling. This enables air to enter the low-ermost part of your lungs and exercises the diaphragm.

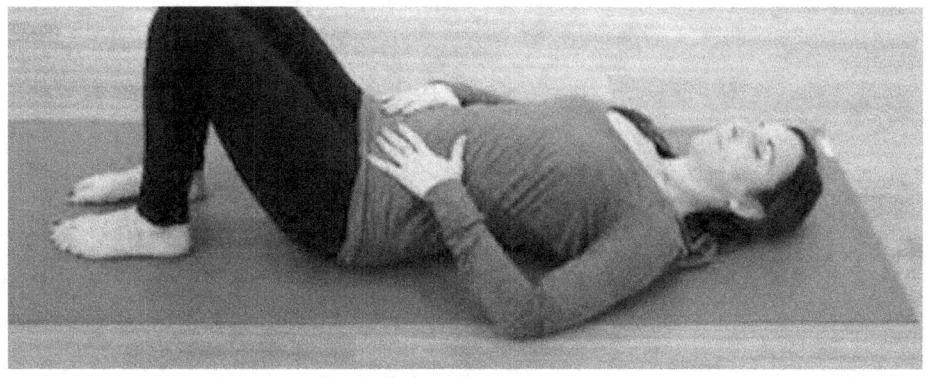

Abdominal breathing[126]

163

The Benefits of Abdominal Breathing

Abdominal breathing is also known as diaphragmatic breathing. The diaphragm is a large muscle located between the chest and the abdomen. When it contracts it is forced downward, causing the abdomen to expand. This causes negative pressure within the chest, forcing air into the lungs. The negative pressure pulls blood into the chest, improving the venous return to the heart. This leads to improved stamina in both disease and athletic activity. Like blood, the flow of lymph (blood minus RBCs), which is rich in immune cells, is improved. By expanding the air pockets and improving the flow of blood and lymph, abdominal breathing helps prevent infection of the lungs and other tissues. Most of all it is an excellent way to stimulate the relaxation response that reduces tension and brings an overall sense of well-being.

Abdominal Breathing Technique

Breathing exercises such as this one should be done twice a day, whenever you find your mind dwelling on upsetting thoughts, or when you are experiencing pain.

- Lie on your back with legs folded at the knees.
- Place both hands on your on your abdomen. When you take a deep breath in, your hands on your abdomen should rise. This ensures that the diaphragm is pulling air into the base of the lungs.
- After exhaling through the mouth, take a slow, deep breath in through your nose, imagining that you are sucking in all the air in the room, and hold it for a count of seven (or as long as you are able, not exceeding seven).
- Slowly exhale through your mouth for a count of eight. As the air is released in a relaxed manner, gently contract your abdominal muscles to evacuate the air

from your lungs completely. It is important to remember that you deepen respiration not by inhaling more air but by completely exhaling it.

- Repeat the cycle four more times for a total of five deep breaths. Breathe at a rate of one breath every ten seconds (or six breaths per minute). At this rate your heart rate variability increases, which has a positive effect on cardiac health.

Once you feel comfortable with this technique, you may want to incorporate words that enhance the exercise. You might say the word *relaxation* with your inhalation and the word *stress* or *anger* with your exhalation. The idea is to bring in the feeling or emotion you want with the inhalation and release feelings you don't want with the exhalation.

In general the exhalation should be twice as long as inhalation.

Abdominal breathing is one of many breathing exercises, but it is the most important one to learn before exploring other techniques. The more it is practiced, the more natural it will become, as it improves your body's internal rhythm.

Use Breathing Exercises to Increase Energy

If practiced over time, abdominal breathing exercises can result in improved energy throughout the day, but sometimes we need a quick pick-me-up. The bellows breathing exercise (also called the stimulating breath) can be used during times of fatigue that may result from driving or when you want to feel revitalized at work. It should not be used in place of abdominal breathing but in addition to it, to increase energy when needed.

This exercise is the opposite of abdominal breathing. Short, fast, rhythmic breaths are used to increase energy, similar to the chest breathing you do when under stress. The bellows breath exercise creates the adrenal stimulation that occurs with stress, and it releases energizing chemicals, such as epinephrine. Like most bodily functions, this exercise serves an active purpose, but overuse results in adverse effects.

Nurture yourself one breath and one small step at a time.

Kapalabhati

Sit in a cross-legged position, keeping both hands on your knees. Inhale deeply, and exhale by rapidly contracting the muscles of your abdomen. Perform twenty-five rapid pumping contractions in each cycle, and do three cycles per day.

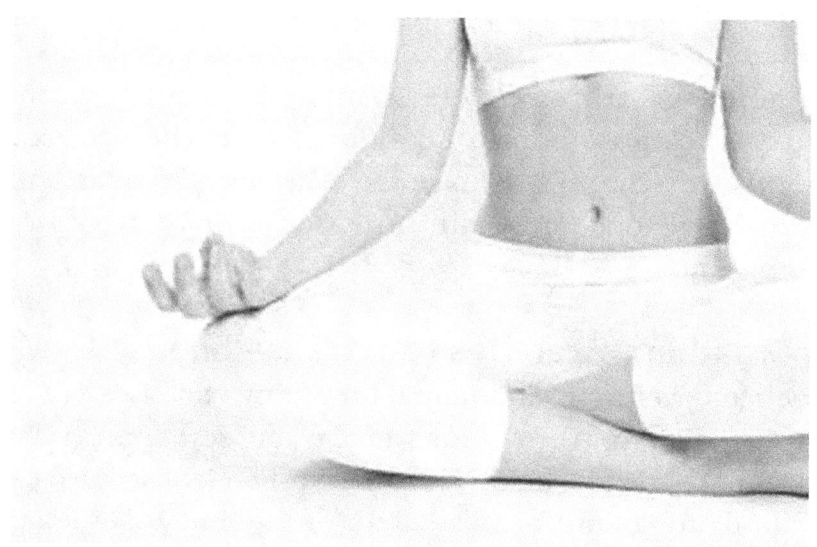

Kapalabhati[127]

Double Leg Lift

Lie flat on your back with your feet together, and keep both hands by your sides. Lift both legs slowly, keeping the knees straight, and inhale while lifting. Lower the legs slowly, keeping your legs as straight as possible, and exhale while lowering. You may or may not lift your head a little. Start with five cycles, and increase to ten.

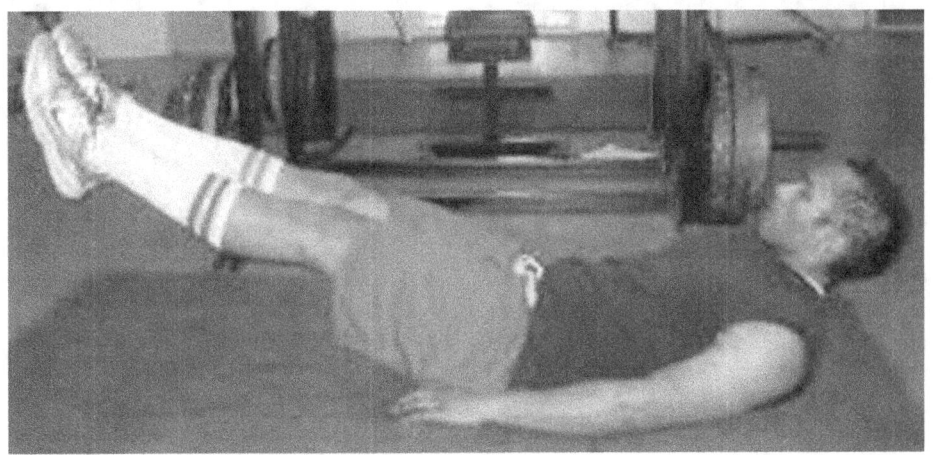

Double leg lift [128]

Forward Bend

This posture helps strengthen the muscles of the spine and the abdomen. More important, it improves the vitality of the organs of the abdomen. It is a head-to-knee posture. Touching your forehead to your knees should not be done forcefully. Do as much as is possible, and you will gradually improve.

Sit straight. Keep your spine straight, and, while inhaling, take your arms up, parallel to your head. While exhaling, bend forward at your hips. Hold your big toes between your thumbs and ring fingers, and try to bring your forehead to touch your knees. Hold the pose for thirty seconds and then stretch up. Repeat three times.

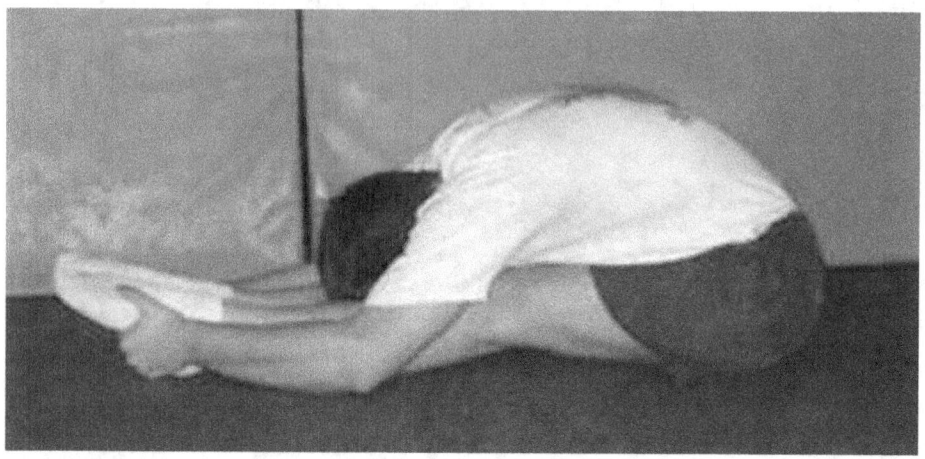

Forward bend [129]

Spine Twist

Sit on the floor with your knees drawn close to your chest. Lower your right leg, and slide it under your left leg. Your right knee should touch the floor, and your right heel should be in front of your left buttock. Lift your left leg over your right knee, putting your left foot on the outside of your right knee. Straighten your back, and turn to the left, putting your left hand behind your right foot. Bring your right arm under your left leg, and hold your left hand at the back. Repeat the steps on the other side; this forms one cycle. Start with one cycle and increase to three. Some poses are difficult and may be done with the help of a trainer.

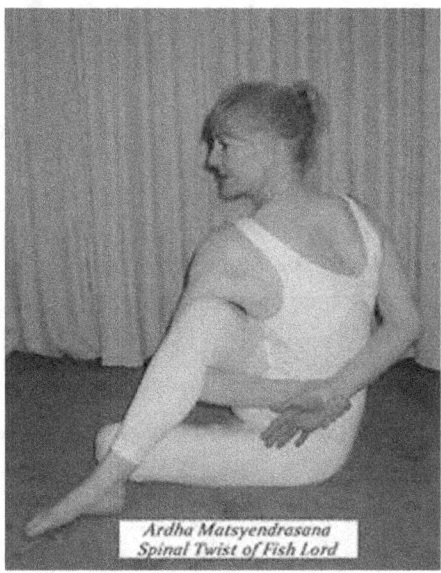

Spine twist [130]

Regular practice of this asana increases flexibility of the spine.

Anaerobic exercises are active, and physical exertion requires extra oxygen to sustain the activity. During these movements the heart rate and breathing increase to keep up with the extra oxygen demand on the muscles. These include brisk walking, running, jogging, swimming, and cycling. (These should not be undertaken without the advice of your treating doctor.) Your pulse rate should never be allowed to exceed 75 percent of 220 minus your age. For example, if you are sixty years old, 220 minus 60 is 160, and 75 percent of 160 is 120, so your pulse rate should not exceed 120.

In these activities the energy needed is derived from the anaerobic metabolic pathway. Lactic acid is formed, and it accumulates in the muscles. As the activity ceases, the negative balance of oxygen is restored, and lactic acid is metabolized.

Aerobic exercises do not require an extra load of oxygen and therefore do not put extra stress on the heart and lungs. These include static cycling, walking on a treadmill, weight lifting, and similar exercises in a gym. [131]

The exercises do not need to be intensive to be beneficial. If you are diabetic, exercise can produce hypoglycemia, so it is essential to have a snack, such as a candy bar, always available. Exercise can also cause rebound hyperglycemia. In such a situation your blood sugar must be estimated. Make the necessary adjustments to your intake of food and drugs.

How much exercise is required? How hard should you exercise and for how long? The best person to monitor your exercise is you. Heart rate and fatigue levels are easy parameters to depend upon. What is moderate for one person may prove strenuous for another, so it is wise to do the workout that agrees with you. It is better to start at a lower level, and, as the body adapts, you can gradually increase the effort. Only you can determine how hard an exercise to start with and the rate at which to increase the effort. The total exercise recommended per day is about an hour, including moderate exercise for more than half an hour. Vigorous exertion should not exceed twenty minutes. Build up gradually.

Walking is one of the best forms of exercise, especially when undertaken early in the morning. Brisk walking sets up the blood-pumping action in the calf muscles and is considered one of the best ways to exercise the heart. Bones stay fit and maintain their strength and density by working against gravity. Jogging and squash are now considered the worst forms of strenuous exercise because the speed of blood circulation increases, and this speeds up arteriosclerosis in the vessels.

To sum up, exercise has the following benefits:
- It increases muscle strength, stamina, and flexibility.
- It increases the power of the heart muscle.
- It keeps the metabolic rate high even after the activity is over.
- It helps control body weight.
- It lowers blood sugar.
- It lowers blood pressure.
- It improves body circulation.
- It increases HDL cholesterol levels in the blood.
- It decreases stress and anxiety and elevates mood.
- It increases sensitivity to insulin.
- It improves sleep and minimizes insomnia.
- It reduces the risk of heart attack and stroke.
- It boosts the immune system and improves resistance to infections.

The calories burned doing different types of exercise (for an adult weighing an average of 150 pounds) are given in the table below.

Activity for one-half hour	Calories burned
Brisk walking	160
Running	350
Swimming	130

Tennis	180
Football	220
Dancing, golfing, baseball	130
Sleeping	30
Gardening	100
Yoga	100
Table work	60
Standing	40

When planning your exercise, keep these points in mind:
- Choose a type of exercise that can be done on a daily basis.
- Choose a type of exercise that is safe, keeping in mind the status of the heart and the blood pressure.
- Choose a type of exercise that will not adversely affect any disability you might have.

For example, it is not safe for a person with arthritis of the knee joints to work out on a treadmill because this will further injure the joints. Static cycling is advisable in such situations.

CHAPTER 16

Obesity

Environment exposes what we inherit.
—Rita Malik

Obesity is now a global issue, and we need to fight it with all our resources and effort.

The causes and management of obesity are discussed in the following pages. The mechanisms that control hunger and appetite as well as the role of leptin are mentioned.

I asked my maidservant, Akhtri, a poor widow with four kids, "Why is it so difficult to lose weight?" She said, "Have you ever seen a poor person who is overweight?" That was a hard-hitting truth. Poor people do a lot of physical labor to earn their livelihoods and eat only the bare minimum to survive. They cannot afford the luxury of indulgence.

Obesity is central to the theme of diabetes, especially in NIDDM and IGT, because obese people are forty times more likely to develop diabetes than fit people. Obesity is one of the most common disorders and among the most frustrating and difficult to manage.

What is going on? What is driving the obesity epidemic?

We're eating too many calories. **+** **We're not active enough.** **That's why we're getting fat and sick.**

Management of Obesity

Although a sedentary lifestyle and overeating are two main factors, there is also evidence that genetic factors influence the development of obesity.

Questions of when to eat, how to eat, what to eat, and how much to eat are critical. To do these in an intelligent and scientific manner, it is crucial to understand the biology of hunger.[132]

The Biology of Hunger

Hunger is a powerful biological drive designed to aid in survival. How much you eat is not always a matter of willpower because the hunger drive is both inborn and environmental. The availability and display of delicious food is a trigger that stimulates the brain to turn the desire to eat into the act of eating. Trying to override the basic instinct for nutritional need by dieting can be counterproductive because this may trigger the mechanism that turns on the appetite.

Signals are passed from the brain to other parts of the body. The stomach, the fat stores of the body, the levels of blood glucose, and the endocrine glands play significant roles in this complex network.

The brain is at center stage. It receives messages from different parts of the body, processes the information, and sends instructions. A specific area in the brain, the hypothalamus, contains the appetite center that determines when and how much to eat. When blood glucose levels in the blood fall or when glycogen stores in the liver are depleted, the brain turns on the desire to eat.

The Chemical Messengers That Control Hunger

A neurotransmitter, NPY (a chemical messenger released from the hypothalamus), spurs the desire to eat sweets and carbohydrates. When you skip breakfast, secretion of NPY is increased, and by lunchtime your system is set for a carbohydrate binge. To avoid this situation, it is advisable not to skip breakfast. Stress and dieting are also said to increase NPY secretion.[133]

Serotonin is another neurotransmitter that comes into action when you are full and have eaten your share of carbohydrates. It acts as negative feedback and informs the brain to turn off the secretion of NPY. Whenever the level of serotonin rises, the level of NPY falls, sending a signal to the brain that enough food has been eaten.

Leptin

Douglas Coleman, working in the 1960s, felt that eating is controlled by a factor in the blood, which in turn is controlled by one or more genes. He refused to believe the prevailing view that obesity was a behavior problem; he stuck to his theory and continued to search for the "satiety factor."[134]

Coleman was born in Stratford, Ontario, in 1931. He earned a chemistry degree from McMaster University in Hamilton and a doctorate from the University of Wisconsin. He spent his entire research career at Jackson Laboratory in Bar Harbor, Maine, where he died at the age of eighty-two. Dr. Coleman and

Dr. Friedman shared the prestigious Laskar Award for their work on the ob (obese) gene and leptin.

Jeffrey Friedman at Rockefeller University started searching for the elusive ob gene. Rudy Liebel, at the same university, had also been searching for Coleman's satiety factor and ob gene. Like Coleman, Liebel thought the satiety factor was produced by fat cells. Liebel had worked with experimental mice and with obese and diabetic patients, and he was obsessed with the idea that there was something missing in obese persons: the link that told the body to eat or not to eat. He felt certain that genetics played an important role in determining weight regulation. He found that the BMIs of identical twins were remarkably similar even when they were raised in separate environments. The BMIs of adopted children correlated with their biological parents', not with their adoptive parents'.

In 1986 Friedman and Liebel started their hunt for the ob gene and located four genes. In 1991 a protein molecule that had the making of Coleman's satiety factor, produced in fat cells and coded for by a mutant gene found in obese mice, was discovered. The satiety protein coded by the ob gene was named leptin (the Greek word *lepto* means "slim").

Stephen O'Rahilly at Cambridge University located a Punjabi family, which had migrated to London from India years earlier, with very obese parents and siblings. He found that the family was deficient in leptin production, similar to the obese mice.

Leptin is a cytokine (a protein molecule) secreted by fat stores. When the fat stores are full, an adequate amount of leptin is released. Leptin informs the brain to turn off the appetite mechanism. The reverse happens when fat stores are depleted. The release of leptin from fat stores is withdrawn, and the brain continues to send appetite signals. A gene controls the production of leptin. In certain strains of mice, when the gene becomes defective, production of leptin and signals to the brain decrease, and the appetite is not suppressed, resulting in obesity. When mice are injected with leptin, their weights decrease.[135]

G. Chen and other scientists have done similar experiments on mice by inducing leptin gene therapy.[136]

The ob gene is a defective gene that prevents the production of an adequate amount of leptin. People who inherit this gene are unable to produce leptin even when their fat stores are full. They are unable to send signals to the brain to suppress appetite, and they continue to feel hungry and eat excessively. Just like obese mice, humans with the defective gene are also infertile.

Galanin is another transmitter that is released when fat stores are depleted and need to be replenished.

Cholecystokinin (CCK) is secreted when the stomach is full and a person feels satiated. This induces the brain to turn off the appetite mechanism. It takes the stomach about twenty minutes to get CCK into operation.

Obesity is difficult to treat, but there is no choice in beating diabetes and other health problems linked with obesity. To do this it is essential to learn healthy eating habits.

First and foremost is your attitude and determination to lose weight. When you decide to lose weight, determine your goal. You will have to persevere and keep going no matter what it takes. You will not achieve your goal in a few days; it may take many months. Remember that as you grow older, your muscle mass and bone mass will decrease, and your physical activity may diminish.

Do not eat skimpy breakfasts or miss any major meals. Do not starve. You will rebound and overeat at your next meal.

Here are some tips for losing weight:

1. Eat slowly. This gives your stomach the time to send the message of satiety to your brain.
2. Eat three major meals with one or two snacks in between. Plan your meals so you get adequate calories, nutrition, and fiber in each. No meal should exceed six hundred to eight hundred calories depending on your activity and type of job.
3. Overcome your cravings for sweets and desserts. A craving is a desire to eat based on emotions (unlike hunger, which is based on biological need). It is all in the mind. You do not need the extra calories, which add weight and provide no nutrition.
4. As a snack drink tea or coffee. This helps to ward off hunger pangs. Eating an apple as a snack is a good habit.
5. Take small helpings, and never take a second helping. Never overeat, which sets your stomach at a much higher satiety level. You will eat more to get the feeling of satisfaction and fullness.

6. Eat more fruits and vegetables, and avoid fatty foods, especially those that are rich in saturated fats.
7. Drink plenty of water, and avoid soft drinks and alcoholic beverages.
8. For the obese, overeating as a result of emotional reactivity can be a problem. A study conducted by Michael Lowe of Rutgers University and William Edwin Dodson Jr. of Washington University showed that obese women were more emotionally reactive and more likely to engage in emotional eating compared to women at normal weights.

Anger, stress, and loneliness can be emotional factors that tempt you to eat. Overcome this habit by doing a constructive activity, such as going for a walk or to a gym for a workout.

Losing weight and keeping it off is not easy, but it has so many health benefits that it should become the first priority in your life.

The problem is that we do not keep track of the calories we eat and often indulge in delicious, fatty meals. Eating less means eating fewer calories, and the easiest way to do so is to cut out saturated fats. Fats are the most concentrated source of calories and the least beneficial form of food. Make it your mission to succeed: adopt healthy eating habits, and remain active.

CHAPTER 17

Managing Stress

Knowledge is power, no doubt. Know yourself first.
—Rita Malik

Stress is an elusive phenomenon, and at times it is inevitable. The following paragraphs discuss the generation of stress and how to negate it.

Managing any disease is incomplete without managing stress. Stress is in the mind, and to deal with it we must analyze it from all angles and aspects that impinge on the mind. We must understand the genesis of stress, how it affects the body, and the best ways to cope with it.

Perhaps the only phases of life when we are free of stress are infancy and early childhood, when the mind is void of hate, jealousy, and ego. As the mind develops and grasps the complexity of the society around us, and as we become conscious of ourselves and aware of our needs, we experience stress. Stress management is perhaps the most difficult aspect to deal with because the environmental factor precipitates disease in those who are genetically predisposed. Stress causes the release of hormones that suppress the immune system, making the body susceptible to disease.

Excessive Desire—the Root of Stress

Perhaps the root of stress is desire. We desire wealth, power, and promotion, and we desire to love and be loved. Desire is like a spider's web that entangles and devours.

There is a continuous entanglement in the web of desire and want, and the more we try to get out of it, the more entangled we become.

In this world of cutthroat competition and rivalry, people often suffer from inflated egos. When they view life in its entire perspective, they realize how absurd this is and how foolish it is to burden the mind with such afflictions. It is wiser to free the mind of shackles that cause distress and agony.

How Do We Deal with Stress?

Can we free ourselves of desires and ambitions? If we can do that, we may wonder what life is meant to be. As long as we live, we cannot escape these situations. We have to learn to cope with adversities and adjust. Anger, fear, and anxiety are mere expressions of our inabilities to deal with stressful situations. Alcohol and drugs are no answers—they only expose our weaknesses.

Perhaps the answer to dealing with our problems lies within us. We have to work out the solutions ourselves, and they must be positive and constructive.

There is evidence that the ways we feel and think have tremendous effects on our body functions. Our optimism and positive attitudes determine our well-being to a large extent. Those with positive attitudes and optimism view their misfortunes as temporary setbacks and move forward in life.

The first step is to take personal responsibility for our attitudes and not bear grudges toward others. Once we take an inward journey, passions slowly ease. At this juncture we make commitments to healthy goals. The paths we chose have to be middle paths, and we must have the faith to tread them. We have to find the strength within ourselves to meet the situations.

The Benefits of Prayer

We derive strength for our faith in God, for faith in God is faith in ourselves. One way to pray is to love and respect all God's creations, especially our fellow beings. Pray by reading the Bhagwad Geeta, a Hindu religious book, which has the teachings of Lord Krishna; the Bible; or the Koran. Reading holy scriptures and chanting hymns eases stress. Right karma or deeds are another form of prayer.

The abstractions of the Upanishads empower the mind to view life from a different perspective. Prayer is a great panacea, and the psychological benefits of faith and prayer are tremendous. The body heals, and tranquility settles in.

When we pray, thoughts stream through our minds. These thoughts create positivism that impinges on the yogic realm. Chanting "om" (a mantra) induces a state of total and sublime happiness that comes only with total detachment from earthly materialism. In ancient Indian literature, this is known as nirvana.

At times I pray, "Oh God, take me into that realm of tranquility where the shackles of materialism do not stifle the soul, where the clarity of thought is not shrouded by hatred and jealousy, and where realization is not made blunt by inferiority or superiority." At that moment I am reminded of a verse written by Nobel laureate Rabindranath Tagore: "O God, wake my countrymen into that morning where the mind is free and the head is held high," from his book *Gitanjali*.[137]

While we live in this world, we cannot be totally detached. A great Indian philosopher and the founder of Buddhism, Gautama Buddha, ordained the philosophy of the middle path. On this path we are not so attached to materialism that it becomes an ailment, and we are not so completely detached that we do not fulfill our obligations to the Earth, to which we owe our existence. This is perhaps a more practical approach.

Meditation is a way to relieve stress. It helps us seek and find God. Prayer and good living are paths that lead to enlightenment and to his kingdom. Prayer, especially in deep concentration, bans disruptive and negative thoughts. Yoga helps achieve the same objective because it stills the mind and calms the soul.

The Benefits of Meditation

Meditation has been proven to decrease the secretion of cortisone; this hormone is released during times of stress, and it reduces immunity, raises blood pressure, and damages the tissues. Another hormone released during times of stress is adrenaline. This chemical constricts the blood vessels, reduces the supplies of oxygen and nutrients to the tissues, and compromises the vitality of the tissues. When such a state is sustained, people are predisposed to hypertension or high blood pressure.

During transcendental meditation the repetition of a mantra such as "om" is used to focus the mind. An object or picture can also be used. When starting out practice meditation for twenty minutes twice a day. Later, when you become more proficient and can achieve the same benefit in less time, it can be reduced.

Other Methods to Relieve Stress

Simple procedures like deep breathing, massaging the neck and shoulder muscles, listening to good music, smelling a perfume such as lavender, and eating Siberian ginseng help relieve tension.

Lying in a hot tub or spa for fifteen to twenty minutes goes a long way in alleviating stress. It relaxes the muscles, improves circulation, relieves stiffness of the joints, and opens the pores. It makes you feel good and puts a stop to a hectic regime.

When sadness clouds happiness, watch a funny movie or read jokes that make you laugh. As the saying goes, laughter is the best medicine.

When people are under stress, they fall prey to reactive eating, and overeating must be avoided at all costs. We must eat to live, not live to eat.

CHAPTER 18

Medication

Medication should be the last resort in treating diabetes, but if a doctor prescribes it, do not avoid it. Allopathic (modern) medicines—oral drugs, insulin injections, and combination therapies—are discussed in the following paragraphs. The modes of action of the drugs and their side effects are mentioned.

Medication includes allopathic and Ayurvedic (ancient Indian traditional herbal) drugs. No form of medication should be undertaken without consulting a medical professional.

Certain herbs that have been found to help regulate blood sugar levels can be tried as adjuvants to conventional therapy.

When diet regulation, weight reduction, and exercise do not help in controlling diabetes, allopathic medicines are emphasized. Antidiabetic drugs include oral tablets and insulin injections.

Oral Pills

The first line of therapy is pills. It is much easier to swallow a pill than take a shot, and it is easier to control diabetes with pills than with insulin injections. Therapy should always be instituted at a low dose and gradually increased until the optimum level of control is achieved. When a single therapy fails, a therapy of multiple drugs can be tried (e.g., tablets with injections or different classes of pills).

The four main groups of the oral medicines for treating NIDDM or type 2 diabetes are as follows:

1. Sulfonylureas, which act on the pancreas and increase the production of insulin
2. Biguanides, which act on peripheral tissues to lower the blood glucose level (especially in the liver) and decrease entry of glucose from the liver into the blood
3. A-glucosidase inhibitors, which decrease the absorption of glucose from the intestine into the blood[138]
4. Thiazolidinediones, which increase the entry of glucose from the blood into the peripheral tissues

Sulfonylureas

Sulfonylureas are potent and effective, with relatively few side effects, but they can cause weight gain and hypoglycemia, and, after prolonged use, they may lose their effectiveness.

This group of drugs is not used for type 1 diabetes. There is hardly any pancreatic tissue capable of producing insulin in type 1 diabetes. Because sulfonylureas have little potentiating effect on the action of insulin on peripheral tissues and depend on functioning pancreatic tissue for their activity, they play no significant role for these patients.

Sulfonylureas are most useful in nonobese people with type 2 diabetes. For obese patients with type 2 diabetes, control of the disease is attempted through weight reduction, diet regulation, and exercise. If these measures fail, oral drugs are given. These drugs are also given in severe cases of type 2 obese diabetes. Sulfonylureas are contraindicated in patients with liver and kidney failure.

There are two generations of these drugs. The first-generation compounds are used only in select elderly patients with cardiovascular impairment. This group of drugs is less potent and less likely to produce hypoglycemia, which can prove dangerous in elderly patients with compromised cardiovascular function and can precipitate heart attacks.

Diabetic patients who have failed to respond to the maximum doses of the most-potent first-generation drugs are given the second-generation drugs. They are much more potent and are favored for younger adults. These include glyburide (DiaBeta, Micronase, Glynase); glipizide (Glucotrol); and glimepiride (Amaryl). Besides acting on the pancreas, Amaryl increases the sensitivity of the peripheral tissues to the action of insulin. Amaryl is a preferred drug and is often given in conjunction with insulin. It is not advocated for patients with ketosis and is not given to persons who are allergic to it.

Biguanides

This class of antidiabetic drugs used for type 2 diabetes was introduced in the 1950s. Phenformin was the first compound in this series, but it was soon discontinued because of its association with lactic acidosis. Research led to the development of better products, and the latest compound to be marketed is metformin.[139]

Metformin (also called glucophage) is considered safe and is now often used as the first line of therapy in treating NIDDM.

It acts on the peripheral tissue in bringing down fasting and postprandial blood sugar levels. It acts on the liver to prevent the formation and release of glucose from the liver into the blood. It also helps in increasing the uptake of glucose from the blood by the skeletal muscles and is believed to decrease glucose absorption from the intestinal tract. In some studies it has been shown to decrease blood lipid levels. It has a synergistic action with glitazones (see page 182) in lowering blood glucose levels. This drug causes patients to lose weight.

Metformin is contraindicated in patients with hepatic and renal problems. It should not be given to persons who drink alcohol. The minor side effects reported are gastrointestinal (such as nausea and vomiting). These effects are transient and dose related, and they are present at the initiation of therapy. It is given as an adjuvant to diet alone or in combination with other oral tablets or insulin. It is administered in divided doses.

Alpha-Glucosidase Inhibitors
This group has two products: acarbose (Precose®) and miglitol (Glyset). These drugs lower blood glucose levels by delaying the absorption of sugars in the intestinal tract. They have a major effect on postprandial glucose levels and keep the levels low, thereby keeping the glycosylated hemoglobin low. They are not given to patients taking lispro (Humalog®) insulin. They are contraindicated in patients with hepatic or renal impairment, and they have mild side effects such as flatulence and diarrhea (48).

Thiazolidinediones
These drugs include glitazones as troglitazone (Rezulin) and pioglitazone. Due to its effect on the liver (failure), Rezulin has

been discontinued. Two other products, Actos and Avandia, are related to Rezulin; they belong to this category of compounds and are on the market. These drugs are considered safe and are gaining favor with doctors and patients.[140]

Actos

This drug is available in tablet form and is taken once a day. It can be taken with or without meals at any time during the day. It helps lower blood sugar levels. Its most important feature is that it helps sensitize the tissues to use the insulin present in the body better whether it is endogenous (the body is making it) or exogenous (the patients take it in the form of injections). Actos works by treating insulin resistance, which is an important underlying defect present in type 2 diabetes, by helping the body use insulin more effectively and respond better to the insulin available.

Unlike the sulfonylureas it does not act by increasing insulin production of the pancreas. It may take a few weeks for the effects of Actos to become manifest. It can be combined with other antidiabetic drugs, such as insulin, metformin, and sulfonylureas. Actos is metabolized in the liver, which means it is broken down there and excreted by the kidneys. Hence it is mandatory to test the liver and kidneys to ensure they are functioning normally before starting this drug.

Actos is contraindicated in type 1 diabetes, pregnancy, lactation, ketoacidosis, congestive heart failure, edema or swelling of the feet, liver or kidney disease, and allergy to Actos.

Actos was generally well tolerated by patients on clinical trials, but they reported a few side effects: upper respiratory tract infections, sore throat, sinusitis, headache, and tooth disorder. Weight may increase with the use of this drug.

Repaglinide

This drug acts on the beta cells in the pancreas and enhances the secretion of insulin. It is as effective as sulfonylureas and prevents postprandial hyperglycemia.

D-phenylalanine Derivatives

These act on the pancreas and stimulate the rapid secretion of insulin, which helps control hyperglycemia and reduce the increase in blood glucose levels that occur after eating. Starlix is one of the available brands.

Insulin

This medicine is given as an injection. It is imperative in treating type 1 diabetes, in which the beta cells in the pancreas cannot produce insulin. It is also indicated for nonobese patients with type 2 diabetes when hyperglycemia fails to respond to diet therapy alone or in combination with oral antidiabetic drugs. Insulin is administered during pregnancy to diabetic women. A diabetic patient undergoing surgical intervention also needs to be put on insulin.

Available insulin preparations differ with respect to the animal species from which they are obtained, their degree of purity and solubility, and the time of onset and duration of action. Insulin preparations obtained from animals other than human beings have the disadvantage of causing allergic reactions because they are foreign proteins. With the availability of highly purified human insulin, the complications associated with insulin injection have reduced considerably. The incidences of insulin allergy, immunity, and resistance have decreased. Human insulin is currently prepared by recombinant DNA techniques, which is a biosynthetic method.

Commercial insulin preparations now available are mainly of the following types:

1. Regular insulin is short acting. When injected, the action starts within thirty to sixty minutes and lasts for five to eight hours. It is a clear, crystalline preparation, and its intravenous infusion is preferred for treating acute diabetic complications as severe infections. It is also used during operations.

2. NPH insulin is intermediate acting. The onset of action is about two to four hours, and the duration of action is about eighteen to twenty-four hours. Lente insulin is also intermediate acting.

3. Ultralente insulin is long acting. The action starts in six to eight hours and lasts for twenty-four to thirty hours.

4. Lispro (Humalog®) is rapid-acting insulin and must be given no more than ten to fifteen minutes before eating.[141]

5. Long-acting insulin called glargine (Lantus) has recently become available. It is taken once a day. It can be combined with short-acting insulin for optimum control of diabetes.

It is customary to combine short-acting with long-acting insulin before and after meals to allow daylong coverage. Stable, premixed preparations containing different concentrations of different types of insulin are available.

Insulin vials should be stored in the refrigerator (not in the freezer) when not in use to avoid loss of medicinal activity.

Site of Injection

The injection is given subcutaneously on any part of the body covered by loose skin. The injection site should be changed periodically because injection at the same site results in fibrosis and lipohypertrophy, which delays insulin absorption. Convenient sites for insulin injections include the subcutaneous tissue of the abdomen, upper thighs, and upper arms.

Methods of Injection

The method of injection depends on the delivery system, which can vary from a simple syringe and needle to insulin pens and pumps.

Disposable plastic syringes with attached needles are available in 1 ml, 0.5 ml, and 0.3 ml sizes. When low doses of insulin are prescribed, it is convenient to use a 0.5 ml or 0.3 ml size because this facilitates more accurate measurement. Disposable syringes can be reused until the needles become blunt. The needles can be used three to five times without compromising sterility by covering them with caps between uses.

Insulin pens are convenient devices that can be used in place of syringes and needles. These are useful for patients with poor eyesight or shaky hands. Reusable pens fitted with cartridges are available and permit quick, easy administration of accurate doses.

Victoza®

This is a new drug that is taken once a day, but it has the serious side effect of pancreatitis.

CHAPTER 19

Home Remedies

Many years of experience and research have gone into the development and use of these preparations. Most are mild and have no side effects, but no medication should be taken without consulting a professional.

Before the development of the modern drug industry, household remedies were used; they have been used on the Indian subcontinent dating back to the Aryan period. Because diet regulation is an integral part of managing diabetes, these remedies are helpful, and they are derived from common foods, herbs, and spices.[142]

All these household remedies were and are in common use in India.

Ginger

Ginger is the rhizome of the plant *Zingiber officinale*. It is used widely in India as a household remedy, and it is one of the basic ingredients in Indian cooking. Preliminary research, carried out in alloxan-induced diabetic rats and rabbits, showed that the administration of freshly extracted ginger juice lowered blood glucose significantly in these animals. Alloxan is a chemical that destroys beta cells in the pancreas and produces diabetes in experimental animals.

Indian Gooseberry

The Indian name is *amla,* and the botanical name is *Emblica officinalis.* Amla is rich in vitamin C. A tablespoonful of its juice mixed with a cup of bitter gourd juice, taken daily, is said to help stimulate the islets of Langerhans. Amla powder mixed with jamun powder and bitter gourd powder is also effective in managing diabetes.

Jamun Fruit

This fruit is called *jamun* in Hindi and Java plum in the English language. The botanical name is *Syzgium cumini.* The whole fruit, especially the seeds, is considered useful in tackling diabetes because of its stimulating effect on the pancreas. In the Aryan period, the bark of the jamun tree was used to treat diabetes.

Bitter Gourd, or Plant Insulin

The Indian name is *karela,* and the botanical name is *Momordica charantia.* In India bitter gourd is considered specific to managing diabetes. Bitter gourd has a compound with insulin-like activity that lowers blood sugar in diabetes. It has many vitamins and antioxidants with many beneficial effects.[143]

Fenugreek

The Indian name is *methi,* and the botanical name is *Trigonella foenum-graecum.*

Fenugreek has soluble fibers called mucilage and other compounds that help lower blood sugar levels and raise HDL cholesterol. According to the Indian Council of Medical Research, fenugreek seeds are highly effective in treating diabetes.

Rebecca Wood has also advocated the use of fenugreek besides bitter gourd, the onion family, stevia, and the sunflower root family.[144]

Lettuce, tomato, and the tender leaves of the mango plant are considered useful and healthy for diabetic patients.

Black Gram

The Indian name is *masha/urad,* and the botanical name is *Phaseolus roxburghi.* It was used widely in ancient times for the prevention of complications of diabetes. Bengal gram, red kidney beans, and mung beans (*Phaseolus munga*) are among the legumes most popularly advocated for diabetics. French beans (*Phaseolus vulgaris*) have been used in India since ancient times for managing diabetes.

Guar

Cyamopsis psoralioides, called *guar* in Hindi, has been one of the most efficient and popular herb used in treating diabetes. Its pods and seeds are used.

Curry Leaves

Murraya koenigi, also known as curry leaves, are widely used in Indian cooking and are considered a good carminative. The infusion of the leaves lowers blood glucose.

Carminatives relieve flatulence, soothe the gut wall, and ease griping pains in the abdomen.[145]

Barley

Barley and barley grass are considered good dietary constituents. They are believed to boost the immune system and help prevent diabetes, arthritis, heart disease, and cancer.

Fruits

Grape-seed extract is a useful dietary supplement because it is a strong antioxidant. It is said to prevent the breakdown of collagen, which is an integral component of tissues.

Aegle marmelos is known as bael fruit in Hindi. The alcoholic extract of the roots and fruits of the plant have been shown to have hypoglycemic activity in albino rats.

The banana is one of the most common fruits in tropical countries. Unripe bananas are considered good dietary constituents for people with diabetes.

Groundnuts

Groundnuts are a rich source of niacin and useful in preventing the vascular complications of diabetes.

Holy Basil

Holy basil is believed to lower blood glucose levels, thereby helping people with diabetes.

Ancient Drugs Used in Diabetes

The following simple drugs were used in ancient times and are still used in Indian households. The Sanskrit terms are followed by the botanical names.

Karavellaka

This is the alkaloid extract of *Momordia charantia*. It produces hypoglycemia and hypocholesterolemia. The effect starts in about two weeks, and it becomes significant in three weeks.

Jambu

This produces a marked reduction of blood glucose levels and brings down blood cholesterol.

Nimba

The Hindi name is *neem*. The leaves are extremely useful in treating diabetes; they are potent hypoglycemic agents and reduce the clotting of blood, thereby preventing vascular complications.

Shilajitu

This has been widely used as an antioxidant and is known for its hypocholesterolemic properties.

Yashada Bhasma

This contains zinc, which helps in the metabolism of insulin.

Loha Bhasma

This contains iron, which helps in the metabolism of insulin.

Gugolipid

This is a derivative of resin from the *Commiphora mukul* tree, and it has been used in India since 600 BC. Indians have used it to treat lipid disorders and alleviate the effects of overeating.[146] This herb, which originated in north central India, is found to decrease blood cholesterol levels. Dr. Szapary of the

University of Pennsylvania studied the effects of the herb in clinical trials in Moradabad, India. He reported decreases of 12 percent in total cholesterol, 13 percent in LDL, and 12 percent in triglycerides.[147]

Madhunashini

Commonly called GS, this belongs to the *Asclepiadaceae* family. It is a wonderful medicinal plant found in India and Africa, and its distribution is now worldwide. Its utility as a medicinal plant has been recognized in Japan and other countries. In India it has been used in Ayurvedic medicine for centuries and is popularly called *gurmar* (*gur* means "sugar," and *mar* means "destroyer") due to its ability to blunt the desire for sweets.

The leaf extract of GS has been used as a remedy for diabetes in Indian traditional medicine. It is believed to have antiviral, antiatherosclerotic, hypolipidemic, and liver-protective properties, and it is said to prevent dental caries. More recently this plant has been picked up by the natural products industries in North America and Europe, and a number of herbal products containing extracts of GS are now available. Experimental studies in humans and animals are being conducted to evaluate its effectiveness in lowering blood sugar levels. In vitro production of the active ingredient in tissue cultures is gaining worldwide popularity.

GS extract is used to treat diabetes in India in various combinations and formulations. It is believed to act in a manner similar to sulfonylureas, to act on the islets of Langerhans, and to boost insulin secretion. It inhibits absorption of glucose from the intestinal tract into the blood, and it decreases the desire for sweets by blunting the sensation of sweet buds in the tongue.

If a patient is on antidiabetic medication, the dose needs to be adjusted when adding GS to the drug regime.

There are many other drugs used in the Ayurvedic branch of medicine, but because documented research has not been performed on them, they are not mentioned here.

CHAPTER 20

Recent Advances in Diabetes

It is always rewarding to keep informed. Some of the recent discoveries in research on diabetes are mentioned in this chapter.

Transplant Surgery

In 1921 Dr. Paul Lacey of Washington University reported that islet cell transplants could cure diabetes in experimental rats. Dr. David Sutherland of the University of Minnesota proved that a patient whose pancreas had been removed surgically could achieve insulin independence by undergoing a transplant of the islet cells.

Trials on Transplant Surgery

It has been a long endeavor to treat diabetes by transplanting beta islet cells of the pancreas, obtained from human cadavers, into patients with diabetes, especially those with type 1 diabetes. Until now the attempts have not proven successful, and several factors have delayed the success. It is difficult to get healthy human islet cells, and there is the problem of rejection of the transplanted tissue. Moreover, the patients have to be kept on strong immunosuppressive drugs, which have potentially dangerous side effects. Research is being carried out to overcome these hurdles.

In one experimental study, islet cells collected from rats were kept in a solution containing alginate.[148] This treatment resulted in creating a hard shell around the cells with pores large enough to allow the passage of insulin and glucose but small enough to prevent the entry of immune cells. These cells were kept in a laboratory, and they were found to generate insulin and respond to changes in glucose levels in the environment. Human trials remain to be conducted.

In May 2000 Dr. James Shapiroal of the University of Alberta reported success in islet cell transplant in eight patients suffering from type 1 diabetes. These patients no longer require insulin. However, they will be kept on immunosuppressive drugs indefinitely so their bodies do not reject the transplanted grafts. The success in these cases has been attributed to a new regime of immunosuppressive drugs. Dr. Thomas Starzl of the University of Pittsburgh (a premier liver transplant researcher) pioneered the use of FK 509, an antirejection drug used by the Edmonton group. The long-term benefits await evaluation.

Although these initial trials are encouraging, it is still to be seen whether these procedures can be carried out in large population.[149,150] The procedure has been done on only a few patients, and the unexpected complications and viability of the grafts are not known.

Research Developments
Scientists have made advances in islet transplantation in recent years. Since reporting their findings in the June 2000 issue of the *New England Journal of Medicine*, researchers at the University of Alberta have continued to use and refine a procedure, called

the Edmonton protocol, to transplant pancreatic islets into select patients with type 1 diabetes, which is difficult to control.

In 2005 the researchers published five-year follow-up results for sixty-five patients who received transplants at their center and reported that about 10 percent of the patients remained free of the need for insulin injections. Most recipients returned to using insulin because the transplanted islets lost their abilities to function over time. The researchers noted, however, that many transplant recipients were able to reduce their needs for insulin, achieve better glucose stability, and reduce problems with hypoglycemia.

In its 2006 annual report, the Collaborative Islet Transplant Registry, which is funded by the NIDDK, presented data from 23 islet transplant programs on 225 patients who received transplants between 1999 and 2005. According to the report, nearly two thirds of the recipients achieved "insulin independence" (defined as being able to stop insulin injections for at least fourteen days during the year following transplantation). However, other data from the report showed that insulin independence is difficult to maintain over time. Six months after their last infusions of islets, more than half of the recipients were free of the need for insulin injections, but at the two-year follow-up the proportion dropped to about one third of recipients. The report described other benefits of islet transplantation, including the reduced need for insulin among recipients who still needed insulin, improved blood glucose control, and greatly reduced risk of episodes of severe hypoglycemia.

In a 2006 report of the Immune Tolerance Network's international islet transplantation study, researchers emphasized the value of transplantation in reversing a condition known as hypoglycemia unawareness. People with the condition are vulnerable to dangerous episodes of severe hypoglycemia because they cannot recognize that their blood glucose levels are too low. The study showed that even partial islet function after transplant can eliminate hypoglycemia unawareness.

Transplant Procedure

Researchers use specialized enzymes to remove islets from the pancreas of a deceased donor. Because the islets are fragile, transplantation occurs soon after they are removed. Typically a patient receives at least ten thousand islet equivalents per kilogram of body weight, extracted from two donor pancreases. Patients often require two transplants to achieve insulin independence. Some transplants have used fewer islet equivalents taken from a single donated pancreas.

Transplants are often performed by a radiologist, who uses X-rays and ultrasound to guide placement of a catheter (a small plastic tube) through the upper abdomen and into the portal vein of the liver. The islets are slowly infused through the catheter and into the liver. The patient receives a local anesthetic and a sedative. In some cases a surgeon may perform the transplant through a small incision, using general anesthesia.

Islets extracted from a donor pancreas are infused into the liver. Once implanted, the beta cells in the islets begin to make and release insulin. However, full islet function and new blood vessel growth associated with the islets take time. The doctor will order many tests to check blood glucose levels after the transplant, and insulin is usually given until the islets are fully functional.

What Are the Benefits and Risks of Islet Transplantation?

The goal of islet transplantation is to infuse enough islets to control the blood glucose level without insulin injections. Other benefits may include improved glucose control and prevention of potentially dangerous episodes of hypoglycemia. Because good control of blood glucose can slow or prevent the progression of complications associated with diabetes, such as heart or kidney disease or nerve or eye damage, a successful transplant may reduce the risk of these complications.

Risks of islet transplantation include the risks associated with the transplant procedure, particularly bleeding and clot formation, and side effects from the immunosuppressive drugs that recipients must take to stop their immune systems from rejecting the islets.

Immunosuppressive Drugs

Rejection is the biggest problem with any transplant. The immune system is programmed to destroy bacteria, viruses, and tissues it recognizes as foreign, including transplanted islets. In addition the autoimmune response that destroyed the recipients' islets in the first place can recur and attack the transplanted islets. Immunosuppressive drugs are needed to keep the transplanted islets functioning.

The Edmonton protocol introduced the use of a new combination of immunosuppressive drugs (also called antirejection drugs), including daclizumab (Zenapax), sirolimus (Rapamune®), and tacrolimus (Prograf). Daclizumab is given intravenously right after the transplant and then discontinued. Sirolimus and tacrolimus, the two main drugs that keep the immune system from destroying the transplanted islets, must be taken for life or for as long as the islets continue to function. These drugs have significant side effects, and their long-term effects are still not fully known. Immediate side effects include mouth sores and gastrointestinal problems, such as stomach upset and diarrhea. Patients may also have increased blood cholesterol levels, hypertension, anemia, fatigue, decreased white blood cell counts, decreased kidney function, and increased susceptibility to bacterial and viral infections. Taking immunosuppressive drugs also increases the risks of tumors and cancer.

Researchers continue to develop modifications to the Edmonton protocol regimen, including the use of new drugs and new combinations of drugs designed to help promote their successful implantation. These therapies may help transplant recipients achieve better function and durability of transplanted islets with fewer side effects. The ultimate goal is to achieve immune tolerance of the islets (meaning the patient's immune system no longer recognizes them as foreign). If achieved, immune tolerance would allow the patients to maintain the transplanted islets without long-term immunosuppression.

Researchers are searching for approaches that will allow successful transplantation without the use of immunosuppressive drugs. For example, one study is testing the transplantation of islets that are encapsulated with a special coating designed to prevent rejection.

Shortage of Islets

A major obstacle to widespread use of islet transplantation is the shortage of islets. Although organs from about seven thousand deceased donors become available each year in the United

States, fewer than half of the donated pancreases are suitable for whole-organ pancreas transplantation or for harvesting of islets—enough for only a small percentage of those with type 1 diabetes. However, researchers are pursuing approaches such as transplanting islets from a single donated pancreas, from a portion of the pancreas of a living donor, or from pigs. Researchers have transplanted pig islets into other animals, including monkeys, by encapsulating the islets or by using drugs to prevent rejection. Another approach is creating islets from other types of cells, such as stem cells. New technologies could be employed to grow islets in the laboratory.

The US government does not endorse or favor any specific commercial product or company. Trade, proprietary, or company names appearing in this document are used only because they are considered necessary in the context of the information provided. If a product is not mentioned, the omission does not mean or imply that the product is unsatisfactory. For information about clinical trials in islet transplantation, see ClinicalTrials.gov or citregistry.org. You may also find information about this topic by visiting MedlinePlus at medlineplus.gov.

Obstructions in Transplant Surgery

The biggest hurdle in transplant surgery is the availability of healthy human islet cell grafts. A team at the University of California, San Diego, recently showed success in developing human beta cell lines that secrete insulin in response to glucose. This development may provide an unconstrained source of beta cells for transplantation, overcoming the shortage of cells from organ donors. Further research will show whether these cells can be safely transplanted in patients with diabetes and whether the cells will produce insulin over long periods.

Stem cell research will open up new avenues of treatment and holds much promise.

Genetic Engineering Research in Transplant Surgery

A gene for islet neogenesis-associated protein (INGAP) may help in changing the dormant cells in the pancreas into active, insulin-producing beta cells. This could benefit patients with both type 1 and type 2 diabetes.

Gene mapping and gene therapy will open up new avenues, and research in this field will provide vast information and valuable clues in the functioning of individual genes. Long-term research in genetic engineering has the potential to develop insulin-secreting human cell lines and techniques of sustaining grafted cells through new immunosuppressive methods, and this could lead to new treatment approaches.

Doctors are now considering pancreatic transplants along with kidney transplants in cases where the kidneys have failed and the only option left is transplant surgery. As the patient has to undergo surgery anyway and live on immunosuppressive drugs, it can be combined with a pancreatic transplant.

Insulin Therapy

Continuing research is bringing innovations in diabetes management. Recent research has focused on developing an insulin inhalation delivery mechanism. This offers a major breakthrough in treating diabetes, but it is still in the experimental stage.

Aradigm Corporation is one of the companies working on developing inhalers that contain the medicine in aerosolized form. This mode of therapy is being used frequently and successfully for managing asthma. However, only a small fraction of the medicine in the inhaler enters the airways, which makes this method of drug delivery expensive. Another difficulty is the delivery of the exact dose, which diabetics must precisely monitor. The insulin used has been of the short-acting type, and efforts are being made to prepare aerosol molecules of longer-acting insulin. Research has shown that insulin can cross the fine membrane that separates the air sacs from the blood vessels in the lungs.[151]

Leptin Injection

Obesity is a chronic disease rather than a behavioral disorder, and it is a major predisposing factor in cardiovascular problems, diabetes, and cancer. Maintaining an ideal weight is crucial in preventing and managing diabetes, so techniques to enhance weight loss may help.

At the University of Texas Southwestern Medical Center in Dallas, scientists injected a recombinant adenovirus, a type of virus,[152] with the leptin gene into healthy rats with normal body fat. The rats overproduced leptin, which resulted in loss of body fat but no lean body mass. Their insulin levels dropped, but diabetes did not develop. It is believed their sensitivity to insulin was directly linked to fat stores. The more fat the body stores, the less sensitivity there is to insulin. These findings may help in understanding insulin resistance in humans. In individuals who have insulin resistance and higher body mass index, percentage of body fat, and amount of abdominal fat, it is possible that their levels of leptin are low or that the brain receptors are resistant to leptin. G. Johannsson's[153] research has shown that humans who are obese and resistant to insulin have higher concentrations of leptin, indicating their brain receptors are resistant to it.

Regranex

Regranex (becaplermin) gel is a recent innovation in the field of biotechnology. It is a cytokine or growth factor derived from platelets (small cells in the blood that help with coagulation). Regranex has been shown to help in healing wounds and ulcers. It promotes proliferation and migration of cells to the site of the wound and helps synthesize new tissues. It stimulates neovascularization (new vessel formation) as well as the formation of connective tissues. The FDA has approved this compound. It is a topical ointment that is applied locally and absorbed through the skin. It is a remarkable adjuvant in treating diabetic foot ulcers, which are serious and, if untreated, can result in osteomyelitis and even amputation.

AGEs

Advanced glycosylation end products (AGEs) are compounds that are formed when blood glucose levels are high and glucose binds with proteins in blood and tissue fluids. They are a kind of glue that seals the pores in the blood vessels and interferes with the nutrition of the cells. AGE inhibitors are now available and used to inhibit or slow the process of combining glucose and proteins, which join to form a complex called AGEs. They do not transform into each other.

Aldose reductase inhibitors (ARIs) are compounds that block the action of an enzyme, which causes accumulation of glucose by-products. They prevent glucose by-products from adhering to nerves and thereby protect the nerves.

Memantine, another drug used in neuropathy, is undergoing trials.

Targretin

Targretin is a compound that has been found to decrease insulin resistance. However, it is still in clinical trials and not ready for use.

C-peptide

C-peptide is a substance normally produced by the body. It is a by-product of insulin synthesis. Its assay in the blood helps estimate the amount of insulin produced. It has been found not only to prevent some complications of diabetes but to reverse them. Administration of c-peptide along with insulin in experimental rats reversed certain complications by nearly 70 percent.

Atorvastatin

Atorvastatin lowers plasma cholesterol by 32 to 38 percent, triglycerides by 15 to 25 percent, and LDL by 43 to 50 percent. It also lowers C-reactive proteins (CRP) and improves endothelial-dependent vasodilatation in type 2 diabetes. CRPs are normally produced in the body and play a significant role in inflammation. Vasodilatation is the expansion of blood vessels.

Endothelial dysfunction is frequently found in diabetic subjects. Diabetic patients have higher levels of CRP than matched nondiabetic controls, and both endothelial-dependent and independent vasodilatation is impaired. Atorvastatin treatment in type 2 diabetics not only decreases the levels of CRP but also significantly improves endothelial functions.[154]

New Drugs in Clinical Trials

Many new preparations that may treat and reverse the ravages of diabetes are in clinical trials.

Byetta, an injectable preparation that mimics a naturally produced hormone, has been approved by the FDA. It is given twice daily. A newer preparation that can be given once a week is undergoing clinical trials. Byetta resembles GLP-1, a hormone produced by the intestine that is believed to promote the growth of new beta cells in the pancreas.

Insulin-sensitizer pills, known as peroxisome proliferator-activated receptor (PPAR) agonists, are being developed by a number of drug-manufacturing companies.

A new class of oral drugs called dipeptidyl peptidase-IV (DPP-IV) inhibitors, which boost the levels of glucose controlling hormones, are also in clinical trials. These drugs also raise the levels of GLP-1.

Acomplia blunts the appetite by blocking brain receptors, and it may prove useful for treating obesity.

CHAPTER 21
Recipes for Diabetics

A healthy diet is imperative for managing diabetes, and diabetic patients need not feel like they are deprived of good food. Many books are available that contain recipes designed especially for diabetic patients. Many food exchanges as well as easy, tasty meal preparations are available. Besides food preparation, portion size, calorie content, and nutritional values are critical elements in day-to-day meal planning.

The following Indian recipes have exotic tastes and are addictive and intriguing. They contain fragrant herbs and rich blends of spices.

Many different blends of Indian spices are available in large supermarkets, like Tops in the United States and in Indian stores or markets. Many of these spices have medicinal value, and some of the preparations given here are recommended in Ayurvedic texts for diabetics. Besides being low in calories, they are rich in fiber and nutrition.

Authentic Indian cuisine gets its distinctive subtle or strident taste by virtue of spices. Ginger, garlic, and turmeric are frequently added. Ghee, which is derived from butter, is used in traditional Indian cooking, although it is advisable to use olive oil or canola oil. Refined mustard oil can be used in certain dishes.

It is best to use nonstick cooking pans because these significantly lower the quantity of fat used. Lentils (*dal* in Hindi) are part of the staple diet in India. *Urad dal*, also known as black gram bean, is used whole or split (i.e., without the skin). *Kala chana* is related to the chickpea but has a brown skin. *Chana dal* is split *kala chana*—without the skin. Other lentils include *toor dal*, frequently used in South Indian preparations, and *mung dal*, also known as green gram.

In the following preparations, the spices can be reduced if a milder preparation is preferred.

Lassi

This is a popular and a refreshing drink. It can be served with or without a meal. It is a favorite drink in summer, as it is easy to prepare, healthy, and soothing.

1 cup nonfat yogurt
¼ teaspoon salt
¼ teaspoon black pepper
Artificial sweetener to taste
Crushed ice

Puree all the ingredients in a blender until frothy, and serve over ice.

Servings: 2
Calories per serving: 60
Protein: 6 g
Fat: 0 g
Carbohydrate: 9 g

Nimbu Adrak Pani

In Hindi a lime is called *nimbu*, ginger is called *adrak*, and water is known as *pani*. This is a refreshing and invigorating drink, especially on a hot summer day.

⅔ cup fresh lime juice
1 tablespoon peeled, chopped fresh ginger
1 teaspoon black pepper
½ teaspoon salt
1 packet of sweetener or 8 tablets of Equal
Crushed ice

Put the ginger in a pan with a cup of water, boil it, and simmer for a few minutes. Strain the mixture into a pitcher; add salt, black pepper, and sweetener, and let it cool. Add lime juice, and stir well. Chill the mixture. Before serving add 4 cups of water, and serve over crushed ice. The calorie content is negligible.

Adrak Elaichi Tea

Ginger is called *adrak*, and cardamom is called *illachi*. This is a refreshing beverage—more so in winter.

4 cups of water
½ teaspoon fresh grated ginger
2 green cardamom pods
Milk or cream (optional)
Sugar or sweetener (optional)
4 tea bags

Put the water in a pan, and bring it to a boil. Add ginger and ground cardamom seeds to the water; cover the pan with a lid, and allow it to simmer over very low heat for 10 to 15 minutes. Strain this into 4 cups, each containing one tea bag. Serve hot. Milk or cream and sugar or sweetener may be added if desired. The calorie content is negligible if no milk or sugar is added.

Servings: 4

Raita

This is a cool, colorful starter. It is quick and easy to prepare.

2 cups nonfat, plain yogurt
1 small onion, finely chopped
2 large tomatoes, cubed
1 fresh green chili, finely chopped (optional)
½ teaspoon salt
½ teaspoon black pepper
1 tablespoon minced or finely chopped fresh mint leaves

Place the yogurt in a bowl, and whisk it until smooth. Add the remaining ingredients, and stir lightly to combine. Cover and chill in the refrigerator until ready to serve. The addition of diced apple, pineapple, cucumber, or cantaloupe can modify this preparation.

Servings: 4
Calories per serving: 80
Protein: 8 g
Fat: 0 g
Carbohydrate: 12 g

Sooji Uppma

Semolina (*sooji* in Hindi) can be used to prepare a number of dishes. It is easy and quick to cook. This is a popular, healthy dish that can be served as a snack or a regular meal.

1 tablespoon cooking oil
1 tablespoon split urad dal
1 tablespoon split chana dal
½ teaspoon salt or to taste
½ teaspoon cumin seeds
½ teaspoon red pepper powder (optional)
½ teaspoon mustard seeds
1 black cardamom
4 cloves
1 small onion, finely chopped
1 cup frozen mixed vegetables or green peas
1 cup semolina
4 fresh curry leaves
Fresh, chopped coriander leaves to garnish

Heat half the oil in a nonstick pan over moderate heat, and add the semolina. Stir gently until the semolina is light brown, and there is a fragrant smell. Put aside. Heat the remaining oil in a separate pan; add mustard seeds, and stir-fry until they crackle. Add both dals, and stir until they are golden brown. Add the remaining spices, and fry for a few minutes. Add vegetables and 3 cups of water, and bring it to a boil. Add the semolina, and cook it over moderate heat until the water is totally absorbed. Garnish with coriander.

Servings: 6
Calories per serving: 200
Protein: 6 g
Fat: 4 g
Carbohydrate: 35 g

Palak Paneer

Spinach (*palak* in Hindi) is a rich source of iron and fiber. *Paneer* is cottage cheese compressed into a cake. It is a rich source of protein with very little fat. In India this dish forms part of a meal that generally includes yogurt, dal, and chapatis (bread resembling tortillas). If paneer is not available, an equal amount of ricotta cheese can be substituted.

2 packages (8 oz. each) frozen chopped spinach
2 packages (8 oz. each) low-fat cheese or a cake of cottage cheese, cut into cubes
1 tablespoon cooking oil or mustard oil
1 teaspoon cumin seeds
½ teaspoon mustard seeds
½ teaspoon red pepper
½ teaspoon salt
½ teaspoon minced garlic

Heat the oil in a nonstick pan over moderate heat. Add the mustard seeds, and fry until they crackle. Add cumin seeds, salt, pepper, and garlic, and fry for about 2 minutes or until the garlic is light brown. Add the spinach and cheese, and cook until the water dries up. A packet of dried *kastoori methi* (fenugreek), about 50 g, can be substituted for garlic. Garlic is a good antioxidant whereas fenugreek is antidiabetic.

Servings: 6
Calories per serving: 80
Protein: 8 g
Fat: 3gm
Carbohydrate: 5 g

Ginger Garlic Halibut

Fish is one of the best forms of protein, and ginger and garlic are antioxidants. This is a healthy, tangy preparation.

4 halibut steaks
1 teaspoon garlic paste
1 teaspoon ginger paste
¼ teaspoon salt
1 teaspoon black pepper

In a small bowl, combine both pastes with salt and pepper. Make fine knife cuts in the fish, and smear the paste into the cuts and all over the fish. Spray a baking sheet with nonstick cooking spray. Wrap the steaks in the baking sheet, putting them side by side. Preheat the oven to 350°F. Bake for 10 to 15 minutes. This method of cooking allows the essential flavors of the fish to be preserved. Serve hot with lemon slices.

Servings: 4
Calories per serving: 130
Protein: 24 g
Fat: 3 g
Carbohydrate: 2 g

Spinach Salmon

Salmon is a rich source of omega-3 fatty acids. Besides having fiber, spinach has high iron content.

4 salmon fillets
1 package of frozen spinach (8 oz.), thawed
1 package of frozen fenugreek (8 oz.), thawed
¼ teaspoon mustard seeds
¼ teaspoon fenugreek seeds
1 tablespoon mustard oil
¼ teaspoon salt
1 teaspoon black pepper
1 tablespoon vinegar

Put the oil in a nonstick pan, and heat over moderate heat. Add the mustard seeds, and heat until the seeds crackle. Add salt, pepper, and fenugreek seeds, and stir-fry until the fenugreek seeds turn golden brown or just a shade darker. Add the spinach and fenugreek leaves; mix the two, and cook for few minutes. Spread the salmon fillets on the leaves. Add vinegar. Cover the pan, and cook for 15 to 20 minutes or until the water dries up and the fish flakes.

Servings: 4
Calories per serving: 280
Protein: 30 g
Fat: 15 g
Carbohydrate: 4 g

Ginger Lime Salmon

Salmon is rich in omega-3 fatty acids. Lime and ginger add good flavors to the preparation. This is a healthy recipe, rich in proteins and long-chain fatty acids.

4 salmon steaks
2 tablespoons fresh lime juice
¼ teaspoon salt
1 teaspoon ginger paste
1 tablespoon butter

Preheat the broiler. Coat the broiler pan with nonstick cooking spray, and place the salmon in the pan. In a small bowl, mix the remaining ingredients. Spread the mixture evenly over the salmon steaks. Broil for 10 to 15 minutes.

Servings: 4
Calories per serving: 360
Protein: 36 g
Fat: 22 g
Carbohydrate: 4 g

Tandoori Chicken

This is a famous Northern Indian preparation. It has a distinctive orange-red color and is cooked in a traditional Indian tandoor (an ovenlike device). This recipe is modified for preparation in a conventional oven.

4 whole, boneless chicken breasts without the skin
½ cup fresh lemon juice
½ cup plain, nonfat yogurt
½ teaspoon salt
1 teaspoon red pepper
1 teaspoon cumin powder
1 teaspoon coriander powder
½ teaspoon cardamom powder
½ teaspoon turmeric powder
1 tablespoon garlic paste
2 tablespoons paprika
1 tablespoon ginger paste
Cooking oil spray

With a sharp knife, make slashes in the chicken breasts about ½ inch deep and 1 inch apart. Rub salt and lemon juice into the cuts, and put the chicken aside in a shallow dish. Put the remaining ingredients in a blender, and blend them coarsely without overprocessing. Rub this marinade into the chicken thoroughly. Place the chicken in the refrigerator, and allow it to marinade overnight.

Preheat the oven to 450°F. Place the chicken on a wire rack in a large roasting pan. Spray oil on the chicken, and cook it in the oven for 20 to 25 minutes or until tender.

Servings: 4
Calories per serving: 300
Protein: 62 g
Fat: 4 g
Carbohydrate: 2 g

Roasted Chicken

This is a quick, delicious recipe. It is similar to the previous preparation but less spicy.

4 boneless chicken breasts without the skin
½ cup fresh lemon juice
½ cup nonfat, plain yogurt
½ teaspoon salt
½ teaspoon red pepper
2 tablespoons tomato puree

With a sharp knife, make slashes in the chicken. Mix all the remaining ingredients except the tomato puree, and rub the mixture over and into the chicken pieces in a bowl. Put the chicken in the refrigerator, and let it marinade for 2 hours. After marinating smear the tomato puree on the chicken breasts, and transfer them to a roasting pan. Roast in a preheated oven at 450°F for 20 to 25 minutes or until tender.

Servings: 4
Calorie content and nutritional values are the same as the previous recipe.

Bitter Gourd

In Ayurvedic texts bitter gourds are considered good for diabetics. The juice extracted from a fresh gourd is effective but bitter, and patients tend to discontinue it because of the taste. Cooked preparations are more palatable. There are several ways to prepare it, and the method described here can be modified to suit individual tastes.

½ pound bitter gourd
1 medium onion, coarsely sliced
1 tablespoon tomato puree
½ teaspoon cumin seeds
1 packet of sweetener
½ teaspoon dried mango powder (*amchor*)
1 teaspoon salt
2 tablespoons cooking oil

Clean, peel, and seed the gourd by making a vertical slit. Smear all pieces with salt, and store them overnight in the refrigerator. Wash and pat dry the pieces, and cut them transversely into ½-inch pieces. Heat the oil in a nonstick saucepan over moderate heat. Add the cumin, and stir-fry for few minutes. Add the gourd, and continue to stir-fry until the pieces turn light brown. Add the onion, and stir-fry until the onion becomes golden brown. Add the tomato puree, sugar, and dried mango powder. Modify the dish by stuffing the long pieces of gourd with mashed potatoes instead of cutting them transversely.

Servings: 4
Calories per serving: 80
Protein: 3 g
Fat: 4 g
Carbohydrate: 8 g

Onion Okra

This is a delicious, spicy dish. The secret of a good preparation is to use fresh, not frozen, okra. This dish is part of the main meal and eaten with Indian bread or chapati.

8 oz. fresh okra
2 tablespoons cooking oil
1 large onion
2 green chilies
½ teaspoon turmeric powder
½ teaspoon salt
½ teaspoon garam masala
½ teaspoon paprika
2 garlic cloves, crushed
1 inch fresh ginger, grated

With a sharp knife, trim the tops of the okra stems, and cut each stem across into ½-inch bits. Cut the onion into long, thin slices. Cut the chilies longitudinally into two halves each. Put the oil into a thick-based, nonstick pan. Add garlic and ginger, and fry for few minutes. Add the onion and okra, and cook over very low heat, stirring gently. Add the spices and chilies. Keep stirring and frying on low heat until the okra becomes soft and tender. Water is not generally added, but if the okra starts to stick to the bottom of the pan, sprinkle with a little water. Serve hot.

Servings: 2
Calories per serving: 86
Protein: 3 g
Fat: 4 g
Carbohydrate: 8 g

Urad Dal

Sabut urad dal, or whole black gram, is a nourishing and popular recipe from Northern India. A lot of butter is usually added, but in this recipe it has been omitted to cut calories and fat. A cup of milk is added to give it a rich taste. Some prefer to add ½ cup of yogurt instead of milk. The addition of green chilies and the generous use of ginger give it a distinctive taste.

1 cup whole black gram
1 tablespoon dried red kidney beans
1 tablespoon fresh ginger, grated
½ teaspoon garlic, minced
½ onion, finely chopped
2 tablespoons cooking oil
Salt to taste
½ teaspoon red pepper
½ teaspoon garam masala
2 fresh green chilies, finely chopped

Soak the beans and black gram in a bowl filled with water, keeping the water level 2 inches above the dal level. Soak it overnight. The next morning drain the water, if any is left. Put the dal and beans with salt in a saucepan. Add 3 cups of water, and cook until the dal is soft and mushy. This can also be done in a pressure cooker. In a separate nonstick pan, heat the oil. Add the onion to the oil, and fry while stirring until the onion is light brown and curls up. Add the ginger and garlic, and continue to fry, stirring all the time, until the garlic becomes light brown. Add the green chilies, and a few minutes later add the red pepper. Add the cooked dal mixture to the fried ingredients. Add garam masala.

Add a cup of milk, and cook over low heat for few minutes. The final preparation should not be too thick or watery.

Servings: 4
Calories per serving: 258
Protein: 9 g
Fat: 6 g
Carbohydrate: 42 g

Red Kidney Beans

All types of beans are rich sources of fiber, vitamin B, and manganese. As detailed earlier, manganese is an important trace mineral required for healthy bones, and it prevents osteoporosis. A diet rich in fiber is essential for proper gut motility; food tends to stagnate in the gut, leading to excessive absorption of cholesterol into the blood—an important risk factor in heart disease. A dish of red kidney beans is healthy and nutritious. Eaten with plain, boiled rice, it is a favorite in Northern India.

2 cups dried red kidney beans
1 teaspoon fresh ginger, shredded
1 teaspoon garlic, minced
1 onion, finely chopped
2 tablespoons tomato puree
2 tablespoons cooking oil
2 fresh green chilies, finely chopped
½ teaspoon red pepper
½ teaspoon garam masala
1 teaspoon salt

Place the beans in 4 cups of water, and soak them overnight. Add 4 cups of water and salt, and cook until the beans are soft and a little mushy. Do not overcook. This may be done in a pressure cooker or a saucepan. Put the cooked beans aside. In a separate nonstick pan, heat the oil over moderate heat. Add the onion, and stir-fry until the onion is golden brown. Add the garlic and ginger, and continue to stir-fry until the garlic turns a shade darker. Add the tomato puree, red pepper, and green chilies, and cook for a few minutes. Combine this mixture with the cooked beans, and add garam masala. Serve warm.

Servings: 8
Calories per serving: 230
Protein: 10 g
Fat: 3 g
Carbohydrate: 40 g

Kaboli Chana

Kaboli chana is like chickpeas. This is another tangy, spicy, addictive Northern Indian dish. It is popularly served with *bhatura*, a kind of deep-fried, puffed bread. When eaten with mango pickle and onion salad, it makes a very delicious meal.

2 cups whole, dried chickpeas
2 tablespoons cooking oil
1 large onion, finely chopped
1 tablespoon fresh ginger, grated
1 teaspoon garlic, minced
Salt to taste
½ teaspoon cumin seeds
1 teaspoon red pepper
1 tablespoon tomato puree
4 pods cardamom
1 teaspoon garam masala
1 tablespoon dried mango powder (amchor)
1 tea bag

Put the chickpeas in a bowl, and add enough water to cover by more than 2 inches. Soak them overnight. Drain the water, if any remains. Put the chickpeas in a large saucepan, and add 6 cups of water. Add the salt and packet of tea leaves, and cook until the chickpeas become soft but not overcooked. Remove the tea packet and put aside.

In a separate nonstick pan, heat the oil on moderate heat. Put in the cumin seeds, and stir-fry until they turn a shade darker. Add the onion, and stir-fry until the onion turns light brown. Add ginger and garlic, and continue to fry. Add a teaspoon of water if the mixture tends to stick to the pan. Add red pepper and tomato puree. Combine the cooked chickpeas with the fried mixture, and cook over moderate heat until the gravy is thick. Add garam masala, amchor, and ground cardamom seeds.

Servings: 6
Calories per serving: 400
Protein: 20 g
Fat: 12 g
Carbohydrate: 52 g

Kala Chana

Kala chana also resemble chickpeas, but they are smaller and have dark-brown skin. They are one of the healthiest foods.

2 cups kala chana
2 tablespoons cooking oil
1 small onion, finely chopped
1 teaspoon ginger, finely chopped
1 teaspoon garlic, minced
1 teaspoon cumin seeds
½ teaspoon red pepper
1 tablespoon tomato puree
½ teaspoon garam masala
Salt to taste
Pinch of asafetida

Asafetida is gum exuded from the root of Ferula, an herb native to Iran and Afghanistan and cultivated widely in India. It is a condiment used along with turmeric in many Indian cuisines to enhance flavor.

Soak the kala chana overnight. Cook them in 6 cups of water, adding salt, until they are tender, and there is a small quantity of water left. In a separate nonstick pan, heat the oil over moderate heat. Add the cumin seeds, and stir-fry until they become a shade darker. Add onion, garlic, and ginger, and continue to stir-fry until the onion becomes light brown. Add tomato puree, red pepper, asafetida, and garam masala. Combine the cooked chana with the mixture in the pan, and serve hot.

Servings: 6
Calories per serving: 260
Protein: 10 g
Fat: 6 g
Carbohydrate: 40 g

Sambar

This is a favorite of both northern and southern Indians. It is a hot, spicy vegetable and lentil stewlike preparation. The basic ingredient is *toor dal* (pigeon peas). Served with rice it forms a staple of the Southern Indian diet. This recipe resembles *sambar*, as it has been modified.

1 cup split toor dal
1 tablespoon cooking oil
Salt to taste
1 teaspoon turmeric powder
½ teaspoon red pepper
½ teaspoon cumin seeds
½ teaspoon fenugreek seeds
½ teaspoon black mustard seeds
¼ teaspoon ground asafetida
6 fresh curry leaves
6 dried red chilies
1 tablespoon sambar masala
1-inch ball of tamarind pulp
2 medium ripe tomatoes, diced
1 medium eggplant, cut into 1-inch cubes
½ pound okra, trimmed and cut into 1-inch cubes

Put the lentils in a nonstick saucepan. Add 6 cups of water, salt, and turmeric powder. Heat to a boil; reduce the heat, and allow it to simmer until the dal is soft and broken. This can also be done in a pressure cooker to save time. Set aside.

Place the tamarind pulp in a bowl, and soak it in a cup of hot water for about 20 minutes. Mash the pulp thoroughly with your fingers; strain through a sieve, and squeeze out as much of the tamarind liquid as possible.

Heat the oil in a large, nonstick saucepan over moderate heat. Add the mustard seeds, and stir-fry until they crackle. Add the fenugreek, cumin seeds, red chilies, and curry leaves, and stir-fry for a few minutes. Add the sambar masala and asafetida. Add all the vegetables, the tamarind pulp, and the red pepper powder. Simmer until the vegetables are tender. Add the dal and continue to stir. Simmer for about 5 minutes. Serve hot.

Servings: 8
Calories per serving: 140
Protein: 7 g
Fat: 3 g
Carbohydrate: 20 g

Punjabi Kadhi

This is a delightful recipe, tangy and spicy, served with boiled rice; it is a favorite in Northern India. It has a yogurt-based sauce with chickpea flour dumplings floating in it. The chickpea dumplings are usually deep-fried and consume a lot of oil, but this recipe is modified—the dumplings have been replaced by onion. Sour yogurt is used in this preparation, but if it is not available, leave plain, nonfat yogurt mixed with a pinch of yeast in a warm place for 6 to 8 hours or overnight. The yogurt will become sour. In place of yogurt, buttermilk can be used.

2 cups nonfat, plain yogurt or buttermilk
⅔ cup chickpea flour
1 teaspoon turmeric powder
1 teaspoon salt
1 teaspoon red pepper
½ teaspoon fenugreek seeds
½ teaspoon black mustard seeds
1 teaspoon cumin seeds
1 large onion, coarsely cut longitudinally
2 fresh green chilies, sliced longitudinally
6 curry leaves
2 teaspoons cooking oil

Place the yogurt in a food processor, and run it for a few seconds. Add the chickpea flour and 6 cups of water, and process to make a smooth mixture.

In a large saucepan, heat the oil over moderate heat. Put the mustard seeds in the oil, and stir-fry until the seeds crackle. Add the fenugreek and cumin seeds, and stir-fry until they darken.

Add the turmeric powder, red pepper, salt, green chilies, and on-ion. Stir-fry until the onions are translucent. Combine the yogurt-chickpea flour mixture and the fried mixture. Bring to a boil, and lower the heat. Continue to stir to prevent curdling. Cook uncov-ered until the mixture is reduced to nearly half its original quan-tity. Add the curry leaves toward the end to preserve their flavor. The dish is ready when the sauce is smooth. Serve hot with rice.

Servings: 6 to 8
Calories per serving: 180
Protein: 16 g
Fat: 4 g
Carbohydrate: 20 g

Sarson Ka Saag

This is a favorite Northern Indian dish. It is eaten with *makka* (corn) *ki roti* (a tortilla-like preparation). Sarson is the mustard plant. It is cultivated in the winter in Northern India and harvested at the beginning of spring. Its seeds are used to prepare mustard oil, and the leaves are consumed like spinach leaves. This is a tasty dish that is rich in iron and fiber.

1 lb sarson leaves
1/2 lb spinach leaves
2 to 3 fresh green chilies
1 small onion, grated
½ teaspoon red chili powder
1-inch piece of fresh ginger, grated
2 tablespoons oil
Salt to taste
1 tablespoon butter

Wash the spinach and sarson thoroughly, and cut them into fine pieces. Cook in a pressure cooker for 30 minutes. Grind the sag, and cook over low heat until it becomes a thick paste. Set aside. Heat the oil in a saucepan. Add the green chilies, onion, and ginger to the oil, and stir-fry until the onion is light brown. Add the sag paste, salt, and red chili powder, and continue to cook on low heat for about 10 minutes. Garnish with butter, and serve hot.

Servings: 4 to 6
Calories per serving: 120
Fat: 4 g
Carbohydrate: 20 g
Proteins 1 g

Sandesh

This is a soft-textured, delicate Bengali sweet made from Indian cottage cheese. It can be prepared with ricotta cheese. It is served as a dessert or an evening snack.

1 pound ricotta or Indian cottage cheese
¼ cup sugar
20 pistachio nuts, thinly slivered

Put the cheese in a sieve and press to remove as much moisture as possible. In a blender process the cheese until it smoothens. Place the cheese in a nonstick saucepan, and heat it gently over low heat, stirring all the time until it forms a solid mass. Remove from the heat, and cool slightly. Add sugar, and mix thoroughly with the cheese. Knead it, and allow it to cool. When cool enough to handle, take small portions of the mixture and roll them into 1-inch balls. Place pistachio slivers on each ball, and place the balls on wax paper. Store them in the refrigerator, and serve them cool.

Servings: about 20 balls.
Calories per ball 57
Protein: 6 g
Fat: 1 g
Carbohydrate: 6 g

Endnotes

1 Http://www.wikipedia.org.

2 Http://www.bing.com/imageshttp://ts1.mm.bing.net/th?&i
d=HN.608024441360550510&w=300&h=300&c=0&pid=1.9&rs
=0&p=0.

3 Alan L. Rubin, *Diabetes for Dummies* (IDG Books Worldwide,
Inc.).

4 Http://ww.bing.com/images/search?&q=elizabeth+taylor+
+images&qft=+filterui:license-L2_L3_L4&FORM=R5IR39

5 Http://ts1.mm.bing.net/th?&id=HN.608039177398389554
&w=300&h=300&c=0&pid=1.9&rs=0&p=0

6 American Association of Diabetes Educators, http://www.
AADEnet.org.

7 American Diabetic Association, http://www.eatright.org.

8 American Diabetic Association. "Nutrition Recommendations
and Principles for the Patients with Diabetes Mellitus (position statement)," *Diabetes Care* 21 (1998): S32.

9 George H. Bell, J. Norman Davidson, and Harold
Scarborough, *Textbook of Physiology and Biochemistry* (The
English Language Book Society and E & S Livingstone).

10 Http://www.bing.com/images/search?&q=Frederick+Ban
ting&qft=+filterui:license-L2_L3&FORM=R5IR41#view=det
ail&id=006A348EC0F6C37E8DF9CF95F1962EFE11AF957B
&selectedIndex=1

11 "Diabetes Statistics," National Institute of Diabetes and Digestive and Kidney Diseases, http://www.niddk.nih.gov/dmstats/dmstats.html.

12 http://www.bing.com/images/search?&q=Global+Diabetes+Statistics&qft=+filterui:license-L2_L3_L4&FORM=R5IR38#view=detail&id=2FA4C6735BB01E0A5182CC0B1351865B9A0505BC&selectedIndex=0;

13 "Diabetes Statistics."

14 American Diabetic Association, "Clinical Practice Recommendations. Management of Dyslipidemia in Adults with Diabetes," *Diabetes Care* 23 (2000): S57–S60.

15 "Data from the 2011 National Diabetes Fact Sheet: Total prevalence of Diabetes," CDC, January 26, 2011, http://www.cdc.gov/media/releases/2011/p0126-diabetes.html.

16 J. Arch and M. Korytkowski. "Strategies for Preventing Coronary Heart Disease in Diabetes Mellitus," *Diabetes Spectrum* 12 (1999):88–94.

17 "Diabetic Neuropathy: The Nerve Damage of Diabetes," National Institute of Diabetes and Digestive and Kidney Diseases, http://www.niddk.nih.gov/health/diabetes/pubs/neuro/neuro.html.

18 American Diabetes Association, "Clinical Practice Recommendations. Diabetic Retinopathy," *Diabetes Care* 23 (2000): S73–S76.

19 American Diabetes Association, "Diabetes nephropathy," *Diabetes Care* 21 (1998): S50.

20 "Diabetic Neuropathy: The Nerve Damage of Diabetes."

21 American Diabetes Association. *Diabetes A to Z.* 1996. April, Ernest W. *Anatomy.* Baltimore: Williams and Wilkins.

22 American Diabetes Association. *Diabetes A to Z.* 1996. April, Ernest W. *Anatomy.* Baltimore: Williams and Wilkins.

23 David Loshak, "Elevated Blood Pressure among U.S. Adults with Diabetes 1994," *American Journal of Preventive Medicine* (2002): 22.

24 Http://en.wikipedia.org/wiki/fileMethane-3D-balls.png.

25 R. K. Murray, D. K. Granner, et al., *Harper's Biochemistry* (Norwalk, Connecticut/San Mateo, California: Appleton and Lange).

26 Http://en.wikipedia.org/wiki/filebenzene-3D-balls.png.

27 Http://en.wikipedia.org/wiki/fileEthane-3D-balls.png.

28 Http://en.wikipedia.org/wiki/filePropane-3D-balls.png.

29 Http://en.wikipedia.org/wiki/filePropanoic acid-3D-balls. png.

30 Bell, Davidson, and Scarborough, *Textbook of Physiology and Biochemistry.*

31 American Diabetic Association, "Clinical Practice Recommendations," S57–S60.

32 Bell, Davidson, and Scarborough, *Textbook of Physiology and Biochemistry.*

33 "Atorvastatin Lowers C-Reactive Protein and Improves Endothelium-Dependent Vasodilation in Type 2 Diabetes Mellitus," JCEM: The Journal of Clinical Endocrinology & Metabolism, last updated July 2, 2013, http://press.endo-crine.org/doi/abs/10.1210/jcem.87.2.8249.

34 Http://www.bing.com/images/search?&q=respiratory+syst em+images&qft=+filterui:license-L2_L3_L4&FORM=R5IR3 9#view=detail&id=BA300721572E29A61C4FBE8B17DAC30 2117AA681&selectedIndex=6

35 Http://www.bing.com/images/search?&q=respiratory+syst em+images&qft=+filterui:license-L2_L3_L4&FORM=R5IR3 9#view=detail&id=BA300721572E29A61C4FBE8B17DAC30 2117AA681&selectedIndex=6

36 B. Cheatham and C. R. Kahn, "Insulin Action and the Insulin-Signaling Network," *Endocrine Reviews* 16 (1995):117.

37 Http://en.wikipedia.org/wiki/fileBilary-system-multilingual.svg

38 Cheatham and Kahn, "Insulin Action."

39 "Herbal Actions: Carminative," healthy.net, accessed September 14, 2014, http://www.healthy.net/Health/Article/Carminative/1471.

40 American Diabetes Association. *Diabetes A to Z*. 1996. April, Ernest W. *Anatomy*. Baltimore: Williams and Wilkins.

41 Juvenile Diabetes Foundation, http://www.jdfcure.com. http://www.aace.com.

42 M. A. Atkinson and N. K. Maclaren, "The Pathogenesis of Insulin-Dependent Diabetes Mellitus," *New England Journal of Medicine* 331 (1994): 1428.

43 W. T. Cefalu, J. S. Skyler, I. A. Kourides, et al. "Inhaled human *insulin treatment* in patients with type 2 diabetes mellitus," *Curr Pharm Biotechnol* (2005): 6387–395.

44 Harvard Health Publication, http://www.health.publication.edu/newsweek/Type of _diabets.htm.

45 Wikipedia contributors, "Asafoetida," Wikipedia, The Free Encyclopedia, accessed September 14, 2014, http://en.wikipedia.org/wiki/Asafoetida.

46 J. H. Karam, "Reversible Insulin Resistance in Non-Insulin-Dependent Diabetes Mellitus," *Hormone and Metabolic Research* 28 (1996): 440.

47 K. S. Polonsky, J. Sturis, and G. I. Bell, "Seminars in Medicine of the Beth Israel Hospital, Boston. Non-Insulin-Dependent Diabetes Mellitus-Genetically Programmed Failure of Beta Cell to Compensate for Insulin Resistance," *New England Journal of Medicine* 334 (1996): 777.

48 Wikipedia contributors, "Insulin resistance," Wikipedia, The Free Encyclopedia, accessed September 14, 2014, http://en.wikipedia.org/wiki/Insulin_resistance.

49 S. Yamashita, et al., "Insulin Resistance and Body Fat Distribution: Contribution of Visceral Fat Accumulation to Development of Insulin Resistance and Arteriosclerosis," *Diabetic Care* 19 (1996): 287.

50 Wikipedia, "Insulin resistance."

51 Yamashita, et al., "Insulin Resistance."

52 Wikipedia, "Insulin resistance."

53 Sivananda Yoga Vedanta Centre, *Yoga: 101 Essential Tips* (New York: Dorling Kindersley).

54 Wikipedia, "Insulin resistance."

55 Yamashita, et al., "Insulin Resistance."

56 "Meta-Analysis of 23 Type 2 Diabetes Linkage Studies from the International Type 2 Diabetes Linkage Analysis Consortium," Karger Medical and Science Publishers, accessed September 14, 2014, http://www.karger.com/Article/FullText/114164.

57 A. T. Hattersley, "Maturity Onset Diabetes of the Young: Clinical Heterogeneity Explained by Genetic Heterogeneity," *Diabetic Medicine* 15 (1998): 15.

58 Carlos Lorenzo, MD, Ken Williams, MS, Kelly J. Hunt, PhD, Steven M. Haffner, MD, *Diabetes Care* 29:625–630, 2006.

59 American Diabetes Association, "Clinical Practice Recommendations. Gestational Diabetes Mellitus," *Diabetes Care* 23 (2000): S77–S79.

60 American Diabetes Association. *Diabetes A to Z.* 1996. April, Ernest W. *Anatomy.* Baltimore: Williams and Wilkins.

61 DCCT Research Group, "The Effect of Intensive Treatment of Diabetes on the Development and Progression of Long-Term

Complications in Insulin-Dependent Diabetes Mellitus," *New England Journal of Medicine* 329 (1993): 977–986.

62 DCCT Research Group, "The Relationship of Glycemic Exposure (HbA1c) to the Risk of Development and Progression of Retinopathy in the DCCT," *Diabetes* 44 (1995): 968–983.

63 DCCT Research Group, "Hypoglycemia in the Diabetes Control and Complications Trial," *Diabetes* 46 (1997): 271.

64 Wikipedia contributors, "Fructosamine," Wikipedia, The Free Encyclopedia, accessed September 14, 2014, http://en.wikipedia.org/wiki/Fructosamine.

65 American Diabetes Association, "Clinical Practice Recommendations."

66 American Diabetes Association, "Diabetes nephropathy."

67 Atkinson and Maclaren, "The Pathogenesis of Insulin-Dependent Diabetes Mellitus."

68 Http://en.wikipedia.org/wiki/.

69 Http://upload.wikimedia.org/wikipedia/commons/a/ae/Circulation_of_Blood_Through_the_Heart.jpg.

70 "Circulatory System," Mrs. Kleczek's AP Biology Wiki, accessed September 14, 2014, http://kleczekbiology.wikispaces.com/Circulatory+System.

71 DCCT Research Group, "The Effect of Intensive Treatment."

72 J. A. Colwell, "The Feasibility of Intensive Insulin Management in Non-Insulin-Dependent Diabetes Mellitus: Implications of the Veterans Affairs Cooperative Study on Glycemic Control and Complications in NIDDM," *Annals of Internal Medicine* 124 (1996): 131.

73 DCCT Research Group, "The Effect of Intensive Treatment."

74 Colwell, "The Feasibility of Intensive Insulin Management."

75 "Atorvastatin Lowers C-Reactive Protein and Improves Endothelium-Dependent Vasodilation in Type 2 Diabetes Mellitus."

76 D. Maron, S. Fazio, and M. F. Linton, "Current Perspectives on Statins," *Circulation* 101 (2000): 207.

77 Scandinavian Simvastatin Survival Study Group, "Randomized Trial of Cholesterol Lowering in 4,444 Patients with Coronary Heart Disease: The Scandinavian Simvastatin Survival Study (45)," *Lancet* 344 (1994): 1383–1389.

78 American Diabetic Association, "Clinical Practice Recommendations."

79 Arch and Korytkowski, "Strategies for Preventing Coronary Heart Disease."

80 Loshak, "Elevated Blood Pressure."

81 Szapary, *Cardiovasc. Drugs Ther* 8[4] (1994):659–64.

82 Maron, et al., "Current Perspectives on Statins."

83 Joshua A. Beckman, MD, MS; Mark A. Creager, MD; and Peter Libby, MD, *JAMA*. 2002; 287(19):2570–2581. doi:10.1001/jama.287.19.2570.

84 "About the 'Metropolitan Life' tables of height and weight," halls.md, accessed September 14, 2014, http://www.halls.md/ideal-weight/met.htm.

85 John Henkel, "Soy: Health Claims for Soy Protein, Question About Other Components." *FDA Consumer* (Food and Drug Administration) 34 (May–June 2000): 18–20. PMID 11521249.

86 "Practice Spotlight: James Rippe, MD, Pioneer in Lifestyle Medicine," American College of Lifestyle Medicine, accessed September 14, 2014, http://www.lifestylemedicine.org/rippe.

87 American Diabetes Association, "Clinical Practice Recommendations."

88 DCCT Research Group, "The Relationship of Glycemic Exposure."

89 Http://www.bing.com/images/search?&q=images+human+eye+ball+verticale+section+&qft=+filterui:license-L2_L3_L4&

FORM=R5IR39#view=detail&id=6E74611900287EEDB37F
E4A1DEFC21207BBF2013&selectedIndex=10

90 American Diabetes Association, "Diabetes nephropathy. "

91 Http://www.bing.com/images/search?&q=cross-section
+of+human+kidney&qft=+filterui:license-L2_L3&
FORM=R5IR41.

92 Https:www.google.com/search?q=STRUCTURE+
OF+GLOMERULUS&client.ww.slumed.edu%252F-
dking2%252Frnguide-htm%3B350%3B279

93 Http://lifeinthefastlane.com/resources/clinical-image-
database/Foot ulcer

94 National Institute of Diabetes and Digestive and Kidney
Diseases, "Diabetic Neuropathy."

95 "Immune dysfunction in patients with diabetes mellitus
(DM)," National Center for Biotechnology Information,
accessed September 14, 2014, http://www.ncbi.nlm.nih.
gov/pubmed/10575137#.

96 P. E. Cryer, J. N. Fisher, and H. Shamoon, "Hypoglycemia,"
Diabetes Care 17 (1994): 734.

97 DCCT Research Group, "Hypoglycemia."

98 Robert Sherwin http://yalemedicalgroup.org/ services/
robert_sherwin.

99 "Practice Spotlight: James Rippe, MD, Pioneer in Lifestyle
Medicine."

100 Nathan D. M., http://carediabetesjournals.org/contents/30/3/753.
long.

101 Anne Maclennam, *N. Engl. J. Med* 2002, 346.393–403: Feb.
7, 2002.

102 Lorenzo, Williams, Hunt, and Haffner, 625–630.

103 Wikipedia contributors, "Asafoetida."

104 Juvenile Diabetes Foundation, http://www.jdfcure.com.
http://www.aace.com.

105 CDC. http://www.cdc.gov/mmwr/preview/mmwrhtml.

106 CDC. http://www.cdc.gov/mmwr/preview/mmwrhtml.

107 "William H. Dietz," Reporting on Health, accessed September 14, 2014, http://www.reportingonhealth.org/resources/sources/William-h-dietz.

108 American Diabetic Association, http://www.eatright.org.

109 "Nutrition for Children," about health, accessed September 14, 2014, http://pediatrics.about.com/od/nutrition/a/nutrition-hub.htm.

110 American Diabetic Association, "Nutrition Recommendations."

111 "Practice Spotlight: James Rippe, MD, Pioneer in Lifestyle Medicine."

112 Therapy of Diabetes Mellitus. Diet and Exercise in Type 2 Diabetes. http://nlm.nih.gov/ftrs/default/browse?hitK=O&search. (1): 42–44.

113 "How can an artificial sweetener contain no calories?" *Scientific American*, accessed September 14, 2014, http://www.scientifi-camerican.com/article/how-can-an-artificial-swe/.

114 "Coenzyme Q10 and Diabetes?" Joslin Diabetes Center, accessed September 14, 2014, http://blog.joslin.org/2011/12/coenzyme-q10-and-diabetes.

115 Jane Kirby, *Dieting for Dummies* (IDG Books Worldwide, Inc.).

116 "Therapy of Diabetes Mellitus. Diet and Exercise in Type 2 Diabetes," http://nlm.nih.gov/ftrs/default/browse?hitK=O&search. (1): 42–44.

117 R. A. Anderson, N. Cheng, N. A. Bryden, et al., "Elevated Intakes of Supplemental Chromium Improves Glucose and Insulin Variables in Individuals with Type 2 Diabetes," *Diabetes* 46 (1997): 1786–1791.

118 L. Jovanovic-Peterson, M. Guitierrez, and C. Peterson, "Chromium Supplementation for Gestational Diabetic

Women Improves Glucose Tolerance and Decreases Hyperinsulinemia," *Diabetes* 45 (1996): 337A.

119 A. Ravina, L. Slezak, et al., "Reversal of Corticosteroid-Induced Diabetes Mellitus with Supplemental Chromium," *Diabetic Medicine* 16 (1999): 164–167.

120 "Coenzyme Q10 and Diabetes?"

121 John Henkel, "Soy: Health Claims for Soy Protein, Question About Other Components," *FDA Consumer* (Food and Drug Administration) 34 (May–June 2000): 18–20. PMID 11521249.

122 Dr. Dunkan Cooper, https://www.google.com/#q=dr+dunkan+of++cooper+institute+in+dallas+for+aerobic+exercises.

123 "Practice Spotlight: James Rippe, MD, Pioneer in Lifestyle Medicine."

124 Sivananda Yoga Vedanta Centre, *Yoga*.

125 Http://jamieonthemat.files.wordpress.com/2010/03/corpse-yoga.jpg?w=500.

126 Http://blissfulwellnesschattanooga.com/wp-content/themes/striking/cache/images/334_Abdominal-breathing1-628x250.jpg.

127 Http://farm9.static.flickr.com/8168/7676579466_42b4fd82d1_z.jpg?zz=1

128 Http://www.bing.com/mages/search?pq-doubleleglift.

129 Http://www.drillsandskills.com/images/stretches/pk001.jpg

130 Http://www.bing.com/images/search?&q=spine+twist+images&qft=+filterui:license-L2_L3_L4&FORM=R5IR39#view=detail&id=69B91BC360DB95E209A8E110AB2D4285E6879F94&selectedIndex=0

131 Dr. Dunkan Cooper, https://www.google.com/#q=dr+dunkan+of++cooper+institute+in+dallas+for+aerobic+exercises.

132 Kirby, *Dieting for Dummies*.

133 Kirby, *Dieting for Dummies*.

134 Coleman Douglas http://gregoryhand1.wordpress.com/ 2014/04/26/the-man-who-showed-that-obesity-is-more-than-just-a-problem-with-self-control/.

135 G. Johannsson, C. Karlsson, L. Lonn, et al., "Serum Leptin Concentration and Insulin Sensitivity in Men with Abdominal Obesity," *Obes. Res.* 6 (1998): 416–421.

136 G. Chen, K. Koyama, X. Yuan, et al., "Disappearance of Body Fat in Normal Rats Induced by Adenovirus-Mediated Leptin Gene Therapy," *Proceedings of the National Academy of Sciences* 93 (1996): 14795–14799.

137 "Where the Mind Is Without Fear," *All Poetry*, accessed September 14, 2014, http://allpoetry.com/poem/8516621-where-The-Mind-is-Without-Fear-by-Rabindranath-Tagore.

138 H. E. Lebovitz, "Alpha-Glucosidase Inhibitors," *Endocrinology and Metabolism Clinics of North America* 26 (1997): 5.

139 M. B. Davidson and A. L. Peter, "An Overview of Metformin in the Treatment of Type 2 Diabetes Mellitus," *American Journal of Medicine* 102 (1997): 99.

140 D. G. Maggs, et al., "Metabolic Effects of Troglitazone Monotherapy in Type 2 Diabetes Mellitus," *Annals of Internal Medicine* 128 (1998): 176.

141 F. Holleman and J. B. Hoekstra, "Insulin Lispro." *New England Journal of Medicine* 337 (1997): 176.

142 Michael T. Murray, *Natural Alternatives to Over-the-Counter and Prescription Drugs* (New York: William Morrow).

143 Bitter Gourd, http://www.stylecraze.com/article/amazing -benefits-of-bitter-melon-gourd.

144 Rebecca Wood, http://www.rebaccawood.com/health/ foods-that-help-prevent-diabetes/.

145 "Herbal Actions: Carminative."

146 Gugulipid http://www.thefreelibrary.com/Traditional+ Remedy+Lowers+Cholestrol++In+Clinical+Trials http://

naturalremediesexplorer.com/remedy-ingreients/gugulipid/.

147 Szapary, *Cardiovasc. Drugs Ther* 8[4] (1994): 659–64.

148 T. Zekorn et al., "Islets cells alginate," *Acta Diabetol* 29:41–45, 1992.

149 E. A. Ryan, "Pancreas Transplant for Whom?" *Lancet* 351 (1998): 1072–1073.

150 A. M. J. Shapiro, J. R. T. Lakey, E. A. Ryan, et al., "Islet Transplantation in Seven Patients with Type 1 Diabetes Mellitus Using a Glucocorticoid-Free Immunosuppressive Regimen," *New England Journal of Medicine* 343 (2000): 230–238.

151 W. T. Cefalu, J. S. Skyler, I. A. Kourides, et al. "Inhaled human *insulin treatment* in patients with type 2 diabetes mellitus," *Curr Pharm Biotechnol* (2005) 6387–395.

152 Chen, Yuan, et al., "Disappearance of Body Fat."

153 Johannsson, Karlsson, Lonn, et al., "Serum Leptin Concentration."

154 "Atorvastatin Lowers C-Reactive Protein and Improves Endothelium-Dependent Vasodilation in Type 2 Diabetes Mellitus."